ETHICS FIELD GUIDE

ACADEMY OF REHABILITATION PSYCHOLOGY

Series Editors

Bruce Caplan, Editor-in-Chief
Timothy Elliott
Janet Farmer
Robert Frank
Barry Nierenberg
George Prigatano
Daniel Rohe
Stephen Wegener

Volumes in the Series

Ethics Field Guide: Applications in Rehabilitation Psychology
Thomas R. Kerkhoff and Stephanie L. Hanson

Ethics Field Guide
APPLICATIONS IN REHABILITATION PSYCHOLOGY

EDITED BY
Thomas R. Kerkhoff
Stephanie L. Hanson

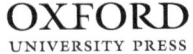

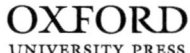

Oxford University Press is a department of the University of Oxford.
It furthers the University's objective of excellence in research, scholarship,
and education by publishing worldwide.

Oxford New York
Auckland Cape Town Dar es Salaam Hong Kong Karachi
Kuala Lumpur Madrid Melbourne Mexico City Nairobi
New Delhi Shanghai Taipei Toronto

With offices in
Argentina Austria Brazil Chile Czech Republic France Greece
Guatemala Hungary Italy Japan Poland Portugal Singapore
South Korea Switzerland Thailand Turkey Ukraine Vietnam

Oxford is a registered trademark of Oxford University Press in the UK and certain other
countries.

Published in the United States of America by
Oxford University Press
198 Madison Avenue, New York, NY 10016

© Oxford University Press 2013

All rights reserved. No part of this publication may be reproduced, stored in a
retrieval system, or transmitted, in any form or by any means, without the prior
permission in writing of Oxford University Press, or as expressly permitted by law,
by license, or under terms agreed with the appropriate reproduction rights organization.
Inquiries concerning reproduction outside the scope of the above should be sent to the
Rights Department, Oxford University Press, at the address above.

You must not circulate this work in any other form
and you must impose this same condition on any acquirer.

Library of Congress Cataloging-in-Publication Data
Kerkhoff, Thomas R.
  Ethics field guide : applications in rehabilitation psychology / Thomas R. Kerkhoff, Stephanie L. Hanson.
  pages cm. (Oxford series in rehabilitation psychology)
  Includes bibliographical references and index.
  ISBN 978-0-19-992807-1
  1. Medical rehabilitation—Moral and ethical aspects. 2. Medical personnel—Professional ethics.
  3. Rehabilitation—Psychological aspects. I. Hanson, Stephanie L. II. Title.
  RM930.K46 2013
  617'.03—dc23
                                     2012048599

Preface

WHEN THIS PROJECT was first proposed, we discussed possibilities, past publications, trends in the literature and our current thinking regarding applied ethics. At first, the focus for the book resided with preparation for specialty board examination—giving the candidate a working model, along with clarifying case examples, to apply in response to ethics scenarios that comprise the oral examination process. However, as happens during the preparation of such works, the perspective broadened regarding applicability in the field of rehabilitation psychology, aiming for relevance across a broad sampling of professional activities in which we engage. Additionally, we had begun to explore in earnest the development of ethics competencies during and after formal training.

The result of this focal broadening is an approach we term a field guide, as one might use to identify different species of animal, plant or insect in the course of observing nature. Our parallel to this model is to structure the book in such a manner that the reader can quickly access cases representing the ethical principles that form the foundation of our APA Ethics Code. We intentionally included case examples within the contexts of varied clinical, educational, and research settings in order to be inclusive of the professional spectrum across which rehabilitation psychologists operate. The intent of our approach is to provide the professional and trainee alike with readily accessible guidelines for parsing out the complexities inherent in applying ethics principles and standards to our wide-ranging work and training environments. Half of the 20 case examples contained in this book are explicated in detail. In these detailed presentations we first present scenarios (critical incidents, in our terminology) that highlight ethical issues, with an invitation for the reader to explore the analysis model we espouse before evaluating the case details. We also include questions before and after each of the case analyses that will enable the reader to delve further into issues raised by the cases. The other case scenarios are briefly presented, along with more limited commentary and a list of relevant ethical standards. These brief case presentations challenge the reader to independently apply the analysis model, identifying relevant contextual features and crafting potential resolutions—a true learning experience. Appended to the book is a list of additional reading and learning resources, designed to provide the rehabilitation psychologist with a representative sample of literature applicable to the field.

The passage of time has also had an impact on this book, as we contrast it to our previous casebook (Hanson, Kerkhoff, & Bush, 2005). Increasing the ease of access to an overview of pertinent issues was a goal that we set out to accomplish. To this end, we include a tabular summary of the detailed case analysis components, along with pro and con statements for alternative case resolutions. Conversely, we wanted to preserve the invaluable aspect of contextual influences on applied ethics conflicts from our previous work in educating students, trainees, and peers, as well as in clinical practice. In our case scenarios, we endeavor to emphasize the decision-making uncertainties inherent in the complexity and ambiguity of events as they unfold; events suffused with realistic character portrayals, simultaneously motivated by uniquely personalized needs and influenced by the social environment. In our experience, it is these uncertainties that most often trigger ethics committee consults within health care organizations.

Thus, the reader can choose a quick reference approach to the detailed cases, or elect to investigate the contextual influences that guided events. In broad strokes, the concept of contextual influences has come to the fore in critical decision-making across a variety of professional settings in recent years (see Roberto, 2009). We see in the evolution of the process of critical decision-making an acknowledgment of the value of contextual factors supporting our conviction that awareness of environmental, biological, and psychosocial contexts offers the professional a more balanced and complete picture of ethical conflicts. In turn, this broad conceptualization of ethical conflicts readily lends itself to applying ethical principles and standards in service of conflict resolution. After all, it is the rich complexity of the course of events across time inherent in human interaction that provides the rehabilitation psychologist with the most intriguing challenges found in everyday professional life.

Thomas R. Kerkhoff, PhD, ABPP/RP
Stephanie L. Hanson, PhD, ABPP/RP
Gainesville, Florida
September 1, 2012

Acknowledgments

WE ARE SINCERELY grateful for the support and academic resources made available through the University of Florida, College of Public Health and Health Professions, and the Department of Clinical and Health Psychology. Additionally, staff support, office space, and professional time provided by Shands Rehabilitation Hospital have been invaluable to the completion of this project.

The complex process of gluing together the disparate parts of this book, organizing the format, checking references, and ensuring that all the pieces are in their proper place (à la APA format) is no small feat. Ms. Katie Sharp must be acknowledged for her yeoman's job of accomplishing what superficially appeared to be an unworkable deed. It is the arcane skills in word processing that members of the clerical profession possess that continue to amaze, and in this respect, Katie epitomizes that profession.

Finally, in the course of generating this field guide, our families must be recognized. Their ability to politely ignore the stacks of articles, books, and notes scattered about our homes was most admirable. In fact, one might say that at times they relished in the chaotic mess representing our unfolding thought process. Yet, that forbearance alone would not have been enough to foster the creative drive to complete this work. Their active support of our endeavors, and understanding of the time commitment necessary to organize and write in service of providing this casebook for your consumption, is much more than simply laudable. We offer our deepest gratitude, respect, and love.

Contents

Introduction, xi

1. Operating Instructions: Decision-Making, 1

2. Principle: Beneficence and Nonmaleficence, 8

3. Principle: Fidelity and Responsibility, 31

4. Principle: Integrity, 52

5. Principle: Justice, 72

6. Principle: Respect for People's Rights and Dignity, 97

7. Conclusion, 118

Chapter References, 120

Additional Readings and Resources, 125

Index, *135*

About the Authors, 143

Introduction

THE TENETS OF bioethics provide foundational guidance for the health care practitioner regardless of discipline, serving to ground professional activities in Western philosophical traditions (Beauchamp & Childress, 2009). These tenets are brought to life when concretized as codes of ethics. All primary health care disciplines have published codes of ethics. Taken collectively, ethics codes provide credible assurance to health care consumers that the health care professionals with whom they interact will reliably demonstrate focal moral virtues—integrity, compassion, trustworthiness, discernment, and conscientiousness (Beauchamp & Childress, 2009). Beyond the basic principles of classical ethics, the Ethics Code of the American Psychological Association (APA, 2002) provides specific, enforceable ethical standards that require adherence by the membership. In addition, the APA Ethics Code (henceforth, the Ethics Code) is episodically revised and updated, incorporating evolutionary societal developments into its principles and standards that reflect current standards of practice. It is this updating process that facilitates currency and relevance in everyday professional life, making the Code a "living process" that guides ethics education and ongoing professional activities within psychology.

Evolving from the Ethics Code, guidelines for assessment and intervention with persons with disabilities have recently been published (APA, 2012). Core values stemming from the ethical principles espoused in the Ethics Code form the foundation for clinical practice and research within rehabilitation psychology. These core values include "respect for human dignity, recognition that individuals with disabilities have the right to self-determination, participation in society, equitable access to the benefits of psychological services, recognition that people with disabilities are diverse and have unique individual characteristics, and recognition that disability is not solely a biological characteristic but is also a result of the individual's interaction with the environment" (p. 44).

COMPETENCE

A core concept embedded in the successful, ethical application of professional skills is competence. Consider your immediate response to the following question: "Do you believe that psychologists should be competent to provide clinical services?" It is likely that you did not hesitate before answering affirmatively, as would almost any other reasonable health care provider. Bush (2007) unequivocally demonstrated this position by stating, "if we do not know what we are doing, we should not be engaging in professional activities" (p. 37). This serves to illustrate that competence is an intuitively appealing concept. However, competence is a much more fluid construct than this answer suggests. Pause for a moment and consider a different question: "Are there circumstances under which it is acceptable for psychologists to deliver care without being competent?" The answer again is a definitive yes. The Ethics Code clearly allows for such circumstances beyond those involved in accommodating student training; for example (and with appropriate caveats) in emergencies and when services would not otherwise be available.

Although the questions above might seem straightforward, inherent in the answers to these questions is the assumption that one understands what competence is. But how do we determine competence to practice? Although standards of competence have been discussed in the literature with increasing vigor over the course of the last half century (APA, 2006), the importance of being able to define and measure competence is particularly highlighted by the 2002 Ethics Code revision, in which competence changed from an aspirational principle to an enforceable practice standard. Competence represents one's knowledge and abilities (knowing how to do something), skills (applying knowledge by demonstrating that ability), and values (appreciating the contextual significance of issues and importance to oneself and others), all operating in the interest of serving others (e.g., delivering rehabilitation psychology care). However, determining the specific knowledge, skills and behaviors, and values consistent with competence is, indeed, a complex endeavor. Consider what application of the competence construct based on the Ethics Code involves:

- Understanding appropriate boundaries,
- Critical skill development in self-assessment (to include evaluating and then applying such knowledge),
- Appropriate judgment regarding seeking training and acquiring skills adapted to the evolving field of practice, and
- Commitment to and actions consistent with consumer protection.

If competence were as uncomplicated as the concept's intuitive appeal, we would not be experiencing a fundamental transformation in clinical psychology education that has been building for years. That is, our profession is essentially moving away from judging a trainee's progression based on numbers (e.g., practica and supervision hours) and moving toward assessment of demonstrated abilities reflecting standards of care.

In addition to the influence of the Ethics Code, and although discussions regarding competence have deep roots in psychology (see for example the 2006 APA task force report), the dialogue regarding competence in the last 10 years has been substantively shaped by the cube model. This model was espoused by Rodolfa et al. (2005) and expanded on by several others. Its intent is to conceptualize and define competencies that would allow measurement of a psychologist's knowledge, skills, and values; thus, it provides benchmarks for educational progression and professional growth and development.

The cube model is a three-dimensional representation of competence, with one axis representing foundational competencies, another axis representing functional competencies, and the third axis representing the professional development of a psychology trainee/psychologist over time. The foundational competencies generally encompass fundamental grounding in broadly applied areas, such as interdisciplinary systems, professionalism, scientific knowledge and methods, and reflective practice and self-assessment. Functional competencies are applied skills and include assessment, intervention, consultation, supervision, research and evaluation, administration, advocacy, and teaching. It is noteworthy that this conceptualization has been adopted by the American Board of Professional Psychology, including the American Board of Rehabilitation Psychology. The developmental axis is tied to classic educational and training milestones—readiness for practicum, internship, postdoctoral training and practice, and ongoing continuing education over the psychologist's career. Specialist training, such as preparation for board certification examination in rehabilitation psychology, encompasses skills, knowledge, and values development beyond the basic foundational and functional competencies. (We briefly comment on this point in Hanson & Kerkhoff, 2011.)

COMPETENCIES SPECIFIC TO REHABILITATION PSYCHOLOGY

Rehabilitation psychology, a recognized specialty within the profession, has a recent body of applied ethics literature with a focus on serving individuals with a wide variety of disabilities (Hanson, Guenther, Kerkhoff, & Liss, 2000; Hanson & Kerkhoff, 2007, 2011; Hanson, Kerkhoff, & Bush, 2005; Kerkhoff & Hanson, 2012; Kerkhoff, Hanson, Guenther, & Ashkanazi, 1997; Kerkhoff, Hanson, & Swaine, 2010) The recent Baltimore conference on developing training competencies in rehabilitation psychology (Stiers, Hanson, Turner et al., 2012) highlighted the importance of skill mastery in applied ethics at varying levels of professional training. While the current movement of competency development and related evaluative processes focuses on training and experience at internship, residency, and specialty certification, it is expected that ongoing ethical maturation occurs throughout the rehabilitation psychologist's career (Hanson & Kerkhoff, 2011). Mechanisms such as mandatory continuing professional education within various state statutes help ensure that the Code remains a nexus of adaptive professional behavior.

Hibbard and Cox (2010) have promulgated competencies for rehabilitation psychologists particularly aligned with the functional competencies at a more advanced level (i.e., in preparation for the board examination in rehabilitation psychology). Examples within the functional competence domain include family's adjustment to disability (assessment), cognitive retraining (intervention), substance abuse management (consultation), and laws related to the Americans with Disabilities Act (advocacy/consumer protection). The 2011 Baltimore conference was another significant step in defining rehabilitation psychology competencies and postdoctoral training site obligations in provision of such training. While each of these steps to delineate rehabilitation psychology competencies is invaluable, we have argued that rehabilitation psychology needs to broaden its focus to encompass predoctoral, as well as postdoctoral competency training (Hanson & Kerkhoff, 2011).

Health care in the United States is strongly challenged by the needs of those with chronic diseases and disabilities. There is much that rehabilitation psychology can contribute to the early stages of one's psychology training to facilitate adequate preparation before graduation to help address these challenges. We provide multiple examples of predoctoral competency issues related to ethics in Hanson and Kerkhoff (2011). In doing so, we have used the Ethics Code as the organizational structure for the ethics foundational competencies, rather than the foundational structure proposed in the competency movement to date. Although ethics has held a firm position in this competency movement, we believe the Ethics Code, with its established history and capacity for adaptation over time, lends itself more effectively as the overarching ethics foundational competency. Whether or not one agrees with this position, ethics is clearly a multidimensional construct. Understanding the layers of training necessary to become competent in the broad arena of ethics is critical to our ultimate goal of facilitating consumer protection and welfare. This book offers the opportunity to highlight situations in which ethical standards come into play during the course of Rehabilitation psychology practice across a variety of health related settings.

Equipping the rehabilitation psychologist with an accessible and relevant applied ethics guide will assist in focusing professional efforts squarely on meeting the needs of the person(s) served. In addition, the quality of professional practice can be enhanced through reliance on the Code's ethical principles and standards as behavioral guideposts during training and throughout one's career. For example, having an applied view can influence multiple domains of service, research, and training, such as crafting and maintaining ethical practice habits, facilitating effective ethical decision-making in individual cases, facilitating effective ethical decision-making within the rehabilitation team process, modeling effective leadership within rehabilitation organizations, creating and refining professional rehabilitation training curricula, and guiding development of rehabilitation research questions and methods that address important issues directly relevant to prospective participants.

RATIONALE

As the reader will experience in the coming chapters, we consider the biopsychosocial model of rehabilitation applicable across many different health related domains. rehabilitation psychologists, imbued with and informed by expertise in the interdisciplinary team approach to health care, often discover a distinct collaborative advantage when interacting with patients, family members, colleagues, and health care organizations—independent of the settings in which they practice. Partly for this reason, rehabilitation psychologists practice across a broad spectrum of health care and research settings. Furthermore, we share the perspective of Rogerson, Gottlieb, Handelsman, Knapp and Younggren (2011), who state, "we believe that ethical reasoning and decision making are not limited to dilemmas, but can be incorporated on a routine basis in psychologists' justifications for all their professional behaviors" (p. 621). Therefore, the case example contexts presented in this book are varied, with the rehabilitation psychologist's collaborative, organic mindset being the common thread linking seemingly disparate issues and settings.

The overall purpose of this book is to offer the reader both an applied evaluative rubric and supporting material geared toward the development of critical analysis skills, and to facilitate efficient and effective decision-making when facing situations with potential ethical implications. While classical ethical conflicts may be somewhat uncommon in everyday practice, decisions made in professional contexts are universally relevant to ethical principles and standards.

Multiple objectives are embodied within the purpose of this book. The first objective is to categorize, within the overarching ethical principles and issues-focused standards, ethical issues encountered in the context of practice, training, and research. A second objective is to provide a decision-making template for the reader by which situations representing ethical issues can be reliably and efficiently analyzed. A third objective is to provide the reader with a choice of using this book as a quick ethics reference resource (utilizing only the critical incident scenario, the analysis table and resolutions for each case example) or as a more in-depth study of the contextual influences on the events of each case example as they evolve across time. A fourth objective is to facilitate ethical principle application by presenting numerous detailed case examples of specific ethical issues (e.g., informed consent, the right of treatment refusal, multiple relationships, etc.) that depict realistic situations. Each of these case examples is analyzed using the template-based decision-making process that facilitates resolution. Additionally, at the conclusion of each case example, we pose several questions to the reader for further investigation that relate to the ethical issue explored in the major case, along with a brief scenario, commentary, and relevant ethics standards for the reader to independently analyze. The fifth and final objective is to provide the reader with a set of reading references to further explore applied ethics issues in the literature, with an emphasis on the field of rehabilitation and the specialty of rehabilitation psychology.

1   Operating Instructions: Decision-Making

CONSISTENT WITH THE broader competency movement in psychology, we believe the process of making efficient and effective decisions when ethics issues arise is a competency that can be developed with adequate guidance and diligent practice using a cogent decision-making process. Bush (2007) cites several decision-making models among many extant in the literature. Some of the models can be applied to ethics issues more easily than others, but the commonalities in all of the models are the following characteristics.

- Gathering information
- Considering alternative solutions and their probable consequences (costs and benefits); along with estimating the magnitude of risk involved in each alternative
- Implementing the alternative estimated to have the best chance of achieving an intended goal and one that is consistent with ethical practice
- Evaluating the outcome of that decision in light of the intended goal

As can be seen in Table 1.1, comparing a number of different ethical decision-making models, a fundamental challenge in any cognitive analysis like decision-making is to appropriately weigh the multiple relevant factors in crafting reasonable alternative solutions. In order to meet this criterion in emotionally charged health care scenarios that raise "red flags" for clinicians and ethics committees alike, the psychologist must take into account the social context and motivational sets of the key stakeholders. Rogerson et al. (2011) offer the following position regarding the nonrational aspects of ethical decision making: "Contextual, interpersonal, and intuitive factors

TABLE 1.1.
COMPARISON OF ETHICAL DECISION-MAKING MODELS

Canadian Code of Ethics (1991)	Koocher and Keith-Spiegel (1998)	Kitchener (2000)	Hanson, Kerkhoff, and Bush (2005)	NASW (2012)
Identify ethically relevant issues	Determine that the matter is an ethical one	Pause and think about response	Identify relevant ethical principles, standards, and conflicts	Determine whether there is an ethical issue or dilemma
Develop alternative courses of action	Consult guidelines available that might apply to identifying and resolving issues	Review available information	Identify relevant organizational and legal concepts	Identify key values and principles involved
Analyze risks and potential benefits of actions on all parties affected	Consider all sources that might influence decision (e.g., prejudices, personal needs)	Identify possible options	Identify context in which conflict has occurred—events leading up to and surrounding the conflict	Rank values or ethical principles most relevant to the issue/conflict, in your professional judgment
Choose a course of action	Consult with a trusted colleague	Consult the Ethics Code	Identify key stakeholders—roles, potential biases, contributions to solution	Develop a plan consistent with ethical priorities central to the conflict
Act with a commitment to assume responsibility for consequences	Evaluate rights, responsibilities, and vulnerabilities of all affected parties	Assess the foundational ethical issues (balance the principles in each option)	Alternative resolutions considered, weighing pros and cons; implement a preferred course of action	Implement the plan, utilizing appropriate practice skills and competencies
Evaluate results of action	Enumerate consequences of possible decisions	Identify legal concerns	Understand case disposition—outcome; adequacy of resolution; are modifications required	Reflect on the outcome of the decision-making process
Assume responsibility for consequences of action	Make the decision	Reassess options and identify a plan		
	Implement the decision	Implement plan and document process Reflect on outcome		

are inextricably linked and inexorably influential in the process of ethical decision making" (p. 616). We proposed a decision-making model incorporating these components (Hanson, Kerkhoff, & Bush, 2005) that has been field-tested by individual rehabilitation psychologists, health care professionals from other rehabilitation disciplines, and institutional ethics committees, with good results (for example, see Kerkhoff & Pugh, 2006).

As will be evident to the reader who progresses through this book, any case example that reflects a realistic unfolding of events will contain ethical elements that typically cut across different ethical principles. Incorporating these different elements into the case analysis is necessary in order to comprehensively explore potential relevant resolutions. Thus, no one ethics analysis model will be the "end-all" for analyzing ethics conflicts. Nonetheless, we have chosen to present our time-tested model in order to provide an overall structure and the conceptual underpinnings for evaluating ethics issues in case scenarios populating the chapters to follow.

The descriptive steps and associated issues of this model are outlined here:

1. **Identifying the Critical Incident**: Health care treatment and research teams face complex decisional challenges on a daily basis, and strong negative emotional valence is often tied to these events. Such complex case challenges and accompanying emotionality can deter individual clinicians, researchers, and treatment teams from efficiently arriving at adaptive decisions. These decisions are often referred back to teams (with clarifying questions appended) by ethics committee consultants that screen consultation requests. In order to effectively work toward resolution, these teams need to clearly identify the critical incident. Critical incidents commonly involve ethical principles and standards but not necessarily ethical dilemmas, and it is important to distinguish difficult clinical and research decisions from ethical challenges. The hallmark of ethical challenges is the presence of at least two ethical principles in opposition. Each of the case scenario examples to follow will open with a critical incident that serves to bring the situation into focus and highlight the ethical issues involved, some of which involve different ethical concepts at loggerheads.

2. **Identifying Ethical Principles and Concepts**: The APA Ethics Code (2002) serves as a core reference in identifying overarching ethical principles and specific standards that apply to a specific situation. The process of utilizing the Ethics Code should become a familiar exercise for psychologists facing ethical challenges in the course of everyday practice. The Ethics Code will not only serve as a tool to clarify the ethical issues at stake, but can potentially help in formulating ethically appropriate solutions. It offers

a coherent conceptual foundation from which to understand the critical incident and can help the psychologist separate an ethical issue from other types of troublesome situations or events, such as managing risk.

3. **Understanding the Social Context and Key Stakeholders**: It is the thorough examination of the biological (health-related), psychosocial and environmental factors influencing ethical issues that places troublesome situations in perspective vis-à-vis problem-solving and decision-making. For example, the rehabilitation milieu and family structure, roles, and dynamics affect perceptions of key stakeholders regarding ethical issues. In addition, each stakeholder involved in the ethical issue has a vested interest in emphasizing a specific perspective that represents personal values and beliefs as they reflect on the target event. Acknowledging the varied points of view during the course of conducting the examination of the contributing factors serves to identify the interpersonal dynamics that fuel such differences of opinion. This examination simultaneously minimizes the likelihood that any key player may become alienated from the process of conflict resolution.

4. **Addressing Organizational and Legal Concepts**: Understanding the medico-legal system of health care in the United States plays an important role in ethical analysis. Federal and state laws and regulations and health care organization policies and procedures can all influence ethics issues and the potential parameters for resolution. Bringing existing legal and organizational concepts to bear on both the contextual factors of the situation and the consideration of alternative solutions can sometimes help the rehabilitation psychologist or rehabilitation team sort through contentious positions. Including these concepts in the process of conflict resolution also acknowledges the vested interest that health care organizations (HCOs) have in minimizing the risk of ethical violations occurring in their bailiwick during the course of health care service delivery (Weber, 2001).

5. **Generating and Anticipating Alternative Resolutions**: At this step in the decision-making process creative problem-solving occurs. There exists the opportunity to take advantage of the rehabilitation team context, with each key stakeholder contributing to the creation of varying resolutions and evaluating probable positive and negative aspects of each alternative. Directed dialogue (in the form of commonly agreed on ground rules) among the players should drive this process, with all ideas initially being considered on merit. Then, consensus-based filtering of alternatives occurs until a primary resolution is identified and implemented. Roberto (2009) states that consensus-building discussions tend to be nonlinear, involving divergence and convergence of ideas in service of making small gains toward an ultimate agreement. In this manner, complex

issues are segregated into manageable components (small agreements) that can then be aggregated in summary. Reaching consensus is a matter of mutual trust. Embedded in this process is the creation of desired outcome(s) attached to the resolution. It is this goal of achieving desired outcomes that the problem-solving effort is intended to achieve.

In each of the case examples, we will detail the decision-making considerations that pertain to each of the alternative resolutions listed in the table. Thus, it should be evident to the reader why any particular resolution alternative(s) were *preferred* within the constraints of the case context. However, the reader is also challenged in each case example to create relevant alternative resolutions not mentioned that might influence the varied dispositions of the cases. In other words, the potential resolutions listed for any case example are not intended to be the universe of valid alternatives worthy of consideration.

6. **Evaluating Disposition**: This final segment of the decision-making process describes the actual outcome of the resolution applied to the situation under consideration. If the actual outcome matches the desired outcome intended by the stakeholders, the process is considered a success. If there is a discrepancy between desired and actual outcomes and the ethical issue remains an impediment to health care provision or the research process the analysis theoretically would revert to the preceding step of the model and other alternatives considered in light of this new information until a satisfactory resolution is reached.

For the purposes of education and utility, in the examples that follow some aspects of the case material are compressed, and tables summarizing pertinent factors considered in crafting resolutions are presented. The reader desiring a brief summary of the ethical issues discussed in each detailed case scenario is instructed to attend only to the "Quick Reference" section of each case. This section includes the critical incident, the resolutions (in italics), and the explanatory table for each case. For those who desire more in-depth information regarding the circumstances of each case scenario, we have focused significant case presentation content on the contextual factors, legal and organizational factors, and resolutions related to the events under consideration in order to bring each case to life. The "Contextual Influences" portion of each case illustrates, in descriptive fashion, the interactional situations in which the case events unfolded, mirroring the complex psychosocial environment that spawned the ethical conflict. Identifying and emphasizing contextual factors affecting ethical issues brings health care practice and research relevance to the exercises.

Following each case example, the reader will find "Learning Opportunities"—questions posed to encourage further investigation of the ethical concepts relevant to the events of the case. Additionally, a brief scenario is presented after each case along with a brief commentary and a list of relevant Ethics Code standards. The purpose of these brief scenarios is to provide the reader with guided opportunities to put the decision-making model to use, exploring ethical issues raised and analyzing the scenarios more fully. An outline of the format for chapters containing the detailed cases is presented below.

Chapter Structure Outline

Principle—Overarching ethics principle from the APA Ethics Code, with explanation
Case Example—identified by chapter and number
Case Title—in *italics*
I. **Quick Reference**—Section of case analysis designated for brief review
   Critical Incident—Trigger event that brings an event to the level of review
   Summary Table—Identified by case example, containing analysis model component information
   Resolutions—Alternative resolutions (in *italics*), along with pro and con qualifiers appended to each alternative; preferred resolution(s) identified
II. **Contextual Influences**—Biological, psychosocial, and environmental factors influencing key stakeholders described in detail
   Commentary—Referenced evaluative discussion of ethics challenges described in each case example
   Disposition—Actual outcome of each case example
   Learning Opportunities—Questions related to the case examples that allow the reader to explore case-relevant ethics issues in more detail, injecting personal perspectives on the material presented
   Brief Scenario—An additional capsule case presentation, offering the reader the opportunity to apply the case analysis model
   Brief Commentary—Guidance provided regarding key ethics issues embedded in each scenario
   Relevant Standards—APA Ethics Code standards related to the ethics issues raised in each scenario are listed to assist the reader in applying the analysis model

The authors take the position that rehabilitation psychologists, exquisitely trained in the interdisciplinary team model of health care provision, are uniquely qualified to offer clinical, educational, and research services both within and outside strictly defined rehabilitation environments. The reader will discover detailed case examples and brief scenarios set outside traditional inpatient and outpatient rehabilitation environments, in which rehabilitation psychologists function competently in providing services to persons in need. It is extensive training in the team treatment process built on core psychology competencies that warrants broadening the definition of the "bailiwick" of the rehabilitation psychologist, extending beyond traditional rehabilitation settings and into the wider health care arena. Finally, the case examples presented in the following chapters represent de-identified, highly modified scenarios based loosely on actual events that the authors have included strictly for educational purposes.

2   Principle: Beneficence and Nonmaleficence

ADAPTING THE ETHICS Code (APA, 2002) definition of beneficence and nonmaleficence, we define this combined principle in the following manner: personal values that reflect the moral obligation to benefit and avoid or minimize risk of harming persons served by rehabilitation psychologists. Looking across the myriad rehabilitation health care disciplines, the bioethical principle of beneficence morally obliges the health care professional (HCP) to act on behalf of person(s) served to render good. There is an expectation of *action* on behalf of that person, and an adaptive moral character on the part of the actor is assumed. For the purposes of bioethical considerations, good is defined as actions that benefit others (Beauchamp & Childress, 2009). Examples of bioethical issues in health care that traditionally fall under beneficence include: rescue, interpersonal reciprocity in helping relationships, actions motivated by quality of life, paternalism, and treatment futility. The latter two examples must be considered in light of HCPs positively disposed to promote good on behalf of their patients. Therefore, beneficence can be served by providing treatment in a paternalistic manner, considered appropriate and necessary (sometimes independent of or counter to patient/family preferences). Similarly, actively avoiding, withholding, or discontinuing treatments (considered futile) that cannot reasonably be expected to provide benefit to person(s) served (sometimes independent of or counter to patient/family preferences) demonstrates adherence to the principle of beneficence.

The bioethical principle of nonmaleficence morally enjoins the HCP to do no harm, along with the obligation to prevent evil or harm and remove evil or harm. The expectation is to intentionally avoid producing a harm, which is defined as thwarting, defeating, or setting back significant physical or personal interests (Beauchamp

& Childress, 2009). Examples of traditional bioethical issues in health care related to nonmaleficence include: rendering (or failing to render) due care, negligence, the negative consequences of interventions gone awry, withholding or withdrawing treatment, ordinary versus extraordinary treatment, the right to refuse treatment, and advance directives. The reader might notice that withholding and withdrawing treatment can fall under both beneficence and nonmaleficence. The differentiating concepts are futility (absence of good), as opposed to administering treatment that is harmful to the patient. Since physical harm is less likely to occur in the realm of psychological service provision, we must consider emotional harm as a morally prohibited equivalent.

It is difficult for the rehabilitation psychologist to imagine professional actions intended to inflict harm or compromise well-being in the context of health care. Indeed, the ethical principles of beneficence and nonmaleficence are essential to our motivational mindset as HCPs. Nonetheless, the complex and varied multidisciplinary health care settings in which we work, and even within the adaptive interdisciplinary treatment teams in which we hold membership, can create social dynamics that occasionally compromise the values and needs of those very individuals to whom we have dedicated our professional lives. Indeed, extraordinary circumstances can arise where compromising good and increasing risk of harm can occur in the course of providing services. It was precisely such circumstantial duress that prompted the APA Council to revise the Ethics Code in 2010 regarding preservation of human rights (APA, 2010).

We now present case examples exemplifying ethical challenges that can arise under the principles of beneficence and nonmaleficence. The reader is invited to critically review the case material, comparing the actions taken by the key stakeholders with alternative approaches not considered. We are reminded that there are many creative, ethically sound pathways applicable to conflict resolution.

CASE EXAMPLE 2.1

"Would you believe it broke again? I'd like to trade it in on a new model."

I. Quick Reference
Critical Incident

In this case example, one of the rehabilitation psychologist's clinical roles is somewhat uncommon, consulting to a solid organ transplant team in an acute care medical center. The psychologist, Dr. Finney, is tasked with evaluating prospective transplant candidates for donated organs and considering selection criteria related to psychological and behavioral status. He is specifically asked for his opinion regarding the possible third kidney transplant for Rena Mulgrew, a 15-year-old who has a history of noncompliant behavior. The social support provided by the patient's mother is compromised because of the mother's relatively poor coping with alcohol abuse and dysthymia. In addition, a distant relative has recently come forward to volunteer as a donor, something the patient and the patient's mother both support as their primary hope to save the patient's life. The findings of the psychological screening factor literally into the life and death decision the transplant team must consider before possible wait-listing and accepting this adolescent for surgery.

This point represents a practical application of how the principle of justice interfaces with the principles of beneficence and nonmaleficence. That is, the rehabilitation psychologist must recommend whether the allocation of scarce resources is appropriate given the patient's psychological and emotional status. Unless benefits and burdens are equal across individuals, the risks and benefits differentially apply, creating the intersection between considerations of beneficence and nonmaleficence with justice. One decision necessarily rules out someone from having access to a scarce resource, at least temporarily, which clearly has associated risks (e.g., waiting longer amid potentially declining health).

Assume that you are the rehabilitation psychologist on this transplant team. Consider the pertinent ethical issues and how you would weigh them in coming to your own recommendation for or against immediate transplantation. Consider the following factors as you weigh your decision:

- What is the emotional integrity of the transplant candidate?
- What is the stability and health of the support system that must be in place after surgery?
- What issues of adherence to behavioral conditions for transplantation are of concern (for example, to the required postsurgical immunosuppressive medication regimen, etc.)?
- Are there any national and organizational policy trends regarding transplants that should be considered?

TABLE 2.1
CASE ANALYSIS SUMMARY

Ethical Principles	Relevant Standards	Context & Key Stakeholders	Organizational & Legal Concepts	Alternative Resolutions
I. Primary Beneficence and Nonmaleficence - Organ transplant teams intend to extend life, and enhance quality of life while balancing costs and benefits - Identification of emotional triggers for noncompliance and associated treatment plan to address family stability may have longer term emotional and physical benefit	2.04 Bases for Scientific and Professional Judgments - RP must be cognizant of current research related to candidate selection and relevance of psychological data to that process 4.06 Consultations - RP must educate the donor and recipient regarding communication of case-relevant information among team members 8.00 Research and Publication - the donor and recipient must be informed about potential involvement in efficacy and outcome research, sharing of identity-protected data with colleagues	- Psychological stability of the adolescent as organ recipient and the family system in predicting sufficient adherence to warrant another transplant - Potential implications of donor's decisional circumstances - Stability of the mother regarding dysthymia and alcohol abuse; impact on daughter's adherence	- "Three strikes" policy implications, if adopted - Health Center's commitment to organ transplant service, responsibility to tenets of UNOS regarding organ prioritization process	A. Approve organ transplant with ongoing support of compliance for recipient and her mother, and careful exploration of donor's motivational set for donation B. Approve organ transplant with a cadaveric donor due to live donor's emotional decision C. Delay approval contingent on patient and family involvement with prescribed interventions
II. Secondary Justice - Team desires to employ equitable candidate prioritization, given scarcity of donor organs Respect for Rights and Dignity	9.03 Informed Consent in Assessment - the donor, recipient, and parent must be informed regarding test purpose and procedures	- RP's role and responsibilities to the patient and the team - Transplant team tasked with equitably prioritizing and supporting appropriate candidates		D. Deny organ transplant due to instability within the family that had resulted in premature organ failure, and may predict future nonadherence

(*continued*)

TABLE 2.1 *(Continued)*

Ethical Principles	Relevant Standards	Context & Key Stakeholders	Organizational & Legal Concepts	Alternative Resolutions
- Adolescent expressed her desire for transplant, and had assented to the procedure, with the support of her mother as guardian				E. Deny organ transplant due to the new "three strikes" policy

Resolutions

    A. ***Approve live donor transplant with support for patient, parent, and donor***

                            Pro

        a) *Transplant approval meets the immediate health needs of the patient*

        b) *Ongoing psychological support meets needs of the patient and mother; likely to increase adherence to immunosuppressive treatment regimen postsurgery*

        c) *Exploration of donor's motivational set intended to avoid negative emotional reaction postdonation.*

                            Con

        a) *Third organ transplant potentially delays other candidates receiving timely treatment*

        b) *Possible negative emotional reaction of donor, given circumstances surrounding decision-making process and possibility of later rejection*

        c) *Potential delayed family guilt and decreased coping regarding live donation if rejection ultimately occurs*

    B. ***Approve transplant with a cadaveric donor—Preferred***

                            Pro

        a) *Meets recipient's immediate health needs; assumes cadaveric match available*

        b) *Eliminates surgical risk for donor*

        c) *Avoids possible negative emotional reaction of donor postsurgery (e.g., if family did not meet her expectations for inclusion)*

                            Con

        a) *Third organ transplant*

Principle: Beneficence and Nonmaleficence

    b) *May not meet family expectations regarding live versus cadaveric donor*
    c) *If rejection occurs, possible regret and/or anger about not using family donor and/or exacerbation of negative coping pattern*

C. ***Delay approval until demonstrated adherence***

    Pro
    a) *Decreases chances of adherence problems, family problems, and emotionality surrounding motivational set for live donation negatively impacting transplantation*
    b) *Timing of transplantation optimized when based on behavioral performance data from psychologist providing patient and family support*
    c) *Retains possibility of live versus cadaveric donor pending evaluative data*

    Con
    a) *Increases health risk for recipient; with possible increase in postsurgical complications*
    b) *Stress on family system increased by delay, despite program support*

D. ***Deny transplant due to nonadherence and familial instability***

    Pro
    a) *Places responsibility for organ failure on recipient nonadherence—predictable behavioral consequence*
    b) *Opens transplant slot for another recipient*

    Con
    a) *Does not meet recipient's immediate health needs; results in chronic dialysis, death*
    b) *Young person with foreshortened life span; could have contributed to society*
    c) *Reduces likelihood of positive behavior change via recipient/family support*

E. ***Deny transplant due to three strikes policy***

    Pro
    a) *Adheres to proposed organizational policy to address overutilization of scarce resources by individuals*
    b) *Places responsibility for organ failure on the patient and family*
    c) *Opens up a transplant slot for another individual in need*

    Con
    a) *Does not meet immediate health needs of the recipient*
    b) *Results in a young person with a foreshortened lifespan*
    c) *Eliminates the possibility of positive behavior change*
    d) *Rigid adherence to such a policy is inequitable; warrants case-by-case consideration*

II. Contextual Influences

Rena Mulgrew is a 15-year-old who is a kidney transplant candidate for the third time. Her first transplanted organ failed almost immediately because of a genetic coagulopathy. The second donated (cadaveric) kidney lasted approximately 10 years, but eventually failed because of inconsistent patient adherence. Rena, having recently moved to Riversend with her family, was admitted to the interdisciplinary transplant team in acute renal failure, stating that she wanted to receive another kidney. Dr. Clive Finney, the rehabilitation psychologist consulting to the transplant team at Riversend Health Center, was asked to evaluate the psychological stability of this teenage candidate. Data from screening evaluations are often predictive of future adherence.

Dr. Finney discovered during his screening that Rena's family system was highly stressed. Rena's father was absent, having abandoned the family several years earlier. Her mother, Chloe Mulgrew, was struggling to overcome a recent bout of alcohol abuse, and had struggled with dysthymia for decades. Mrs. Mulgrew managed adequately most of the time on medication and periodic counseling, but was also prone to episodes of debilitating weekend binge drinking. Chloe Mulgrew was employed as an office manager in a local multispecialty health care practice. She had held a similar position for twelve years prior to moving her family to Riversend. Rena had one older sister, who had left home at 18 years old, and had little to do with the nuclear family. However, she and Rena did e-mail on occasion without their mother's knowledge (a fact divulged to Dr. Finney during the screen evaluation). This protected relationship had little bearing on the current case, except as evidence of Rena's ability to reach out for support to a family member at a distance in lieu of more proximal emotional support.

Rena's nonadherent behavior had resulted in episodes of missed and off-schedule immunosuppressant medication dosing. It was noted by Dr. Finney that many of Rena's episodes of nonadherence coincided with her mother's alcoholic binges. Her pattern of maladaptive behavior was not totally unpredictable, given her adolescent age and history of family stressors, but the consequences were potentially lethal.

As if the case wasn't already complicated, a live donor had entered the picture. Georgia Cane, a distant unmarried cousin of Rena's mother, had lived in the same region of the state since childhood. Learning of Rena's plight, she traveled to Riversend and introduced herself to the transplant team coordinator, emphatically stating that she had been chosen by God (during a recent revival) to become Rena's donor, even though she had never met Rena. Georgia then announced her intentions to the team during a family conference to which she was invited. Rena immediately clung to her distant relative as her last best hope for transplantation. Fortunately, the tissue match was optimal. Chloe too saw her cousin Georgia's willingness to become a live donor as significantly increasing her daughter's chances of survival. The family quickly reached a consensus and demanded to schedule surgery as soon as possible.

Dr. Finney's evaluative team input was critical to the transplantation decision. The Riversend transplant service was considering adopting a rather controversial "three strikes and you're out" policy. This policy stated that candidates applying for transplantation three or more times would be given a low priority. This proposed policy was based on both internal and collaborative transplant center outcome research that had demonstrated negative survivability after multiple procedures. Additionally, organ availability was scarce, live donor procedures were risky, and the circumstances of Georgia's volunteering had highly emotional overtones. Finally, there had been a recent US Supreme Court decision supporting a similarly labeled contingency-based decision-making model in criminal cases.[1]

Commentary

The chronology of this case is pertinent in that a pattern of nonadherence was established in Rena's behavior that contributed in part to the failure of her second renal transplant. While this pattern might lead to a rejection for transplantation, the psychologist must weigh both the factors involved in the nonadherence and his or her influence in "righting the ship." The causative factors influencing this nonadherence are likely several: adolescent rebellion played out, family dynamics influencing the underdevelopment of adaptive compliance behaviors at a young age, and Chloe's chronic dysthymia and alcohol abuse contributing to inconsistent adaptive parenting. Because the issue of patient compliance with an antirejection medication regimen, and adhering to an adaptive lifestyle are central to the transplant team's decision-making process, identifying evidence of potential compliance in Rena's current daily life is important. The psychologist can evaluate this through consideration of issues such as maintaining Rena's hemodialysis schedule, medication usage, avoiding compromising lifestyle behaviors (e.g., prohibited substance use—especially in the presence of her mother's modeled nonacceptable behavior), and complying with the different aspects of the transplant candidacy process. Rena's developmental maturity

---

[1.] This is a modified version of a case provided to the first author by Dr. James R. Rodrique, and originally cited in Rodrigue (2002).

in providing **assent** to these components can offer excellent insight into the structure that also might be needed postoperatively. Though a minor, Rena is at a developmental point where she likely will be able to understand the gravity of nonadherence. Therefore, she can participate in the decision-making process, increasing the likelihood of committing to an adaptive postsurgical compliance regimen. However, because adolescence is characterized by situational actions of reckless autonomy, it is unrealistic to expect 100% compliance even given life and death circumstances that are not immediately apparent. Each of the above factors helps the psychologist weigh the potential risks and benefits of allocating a scarce resource and under what conditions.

The transplant team typically has four options to consider for the United Network for Organ Sharing (UNOS) listing with each candidate:

a) Unconditional listing for available organ
b) Conditional listing, contingent on the patient satisfactorily completing psychological treatment to qualify for listing
c) Delayed listing for a stated period of time, during which the patient is monitored and must demonstrate appropriate and consistent adherent behaviors
d) Not listing, and referral to another transplant program

Given Chloe's role as Rena's parent/guardian, the transplant team might well recommend option b or c; specifically that she seek treatment for her alcohol abuse. She may be asked to provide evidence of her abstinence for a set period of time prior to listing or surgery. This might take the form of written and verbal reports from treating professionals. Chloe, Rena, and Georgia may also be required to engage in psychological treatment with an expressed goal of clarifying family relationship issues impacting transplantation, no matter the final outcome. Involvement in psychological intervention by Rena and her mother will also be a probable requirement of the team. Having the psychologist set up a positive reinforcement system, shaping appropriate family support, as part of treatment to maximize adherence and/or more healthy behavior will likely be a component of any path selected.

Additionally, the circumstances of Georgia's decision to become a live donor (i.e., spontaneous religious motivation in a very short decision time frame) will need to be explored. The team will likely require a thorough psychosocial history, including an assessment of Georgia's motivations for donation, postoperative expectations (e.g., medical recovery, impact on family relationships), and commitment to a healthy recovery process. The commitment of all major stakeholders—Rena, Chloe, and Georgia—to the regimented demands of organ transplantation, both preoperatively and postoperatively, will be a core component of determining whether the benefits outweigh the risks. (See Anbarci & Coglayan, 2005, and Rosner, 2006, for more information regarding live vs. cadaveric organ donation).

Finally, the "three strikes" policy proposal related to this case was in response to concerns expressed at the national level regarding appropriate shepherding of a limited resource, with a goal of extending the potential benefits of solid organ transplant to the most people. It reflected a resource allocation issue that, given broad policy level decisions, could be followed irrespective of individual patient circumstances. However, it is unlikely that such a policy would see rigid adherence, even if adopted as an official national organization stance, given the intensely personal nature of and investment in the relationship between patients and their transplant teams, and the practice autonomy extant at local levels.

Disposition

Rena L. Mulgrew received a live kidney donation from Georgia Cane after 10 days of preparatory intervention with Dr. Finney. Intervention in this case was conceptualized as a layered, sequential process involving both immediate steps to increase compliance and longer term steps to address long-standing family dysfunction. The immediate intervention consisted of motivational interviewing coupled with positive reinforcement, with a focus on reinforcing personal adherence to immunosuppressive medication regimen and regular communication with the transplant team for health monitoring. Once the patient was physically strong enough, the longer term treatment plan included individual therapy to address the patient's poor coping response to her mother's maladaptive behavior and family therapy to address the development of a healthier family environment within the family system dynamic.

The surgery was ultimately tied to Rena's deteriorating medical condition, thus prioritizing near-term nonmaleficence over potential adherence issues related to justice. Fortunately, the surgery was successful and without complications for the patient and donor. After her postsurgery recovery, Georgia took a 12-month leave of absence from work and moved in with the Mulgrews to provide support for the continued health of both Rena and Chloe. At 9-month follow-up evaluation with Dr. Finney, all three reported engaging in family therapy, with a collectively agreed goal of maintaining a consistent pattern of adaptive health behaviors given the gravity of the alternative.

Learning Opportunities

1. Describe the scenario of the rehabilitation psychologist's interaction with the transplant team as he presented his evaluation findings, considering the factors he might have emphasized in making his recommendation.
2. Given the decision to move forward with the procedure, would you have arrived at a different conclusion? If so, identify the factors that would have guided your thinking.
3. Debate whether nonmaleficence should drive transplant decisions with adolescents.

Brief Scenario: Dr. Bob Frederick, a rehabilitation psychologist working in a state correctional facility (medium security), has been asked by the associate warden to supervise the questioning of an inmate allegedly involved in organizing a recent disturbance in the facility in which several staff and inmates were injured. The outcome of this investigation could result in sanctions against the inmate. Dr. Frederick is an employee of the facility, serving as a clinician for the incarcerated population. However, he has also been involved in program development and policy-making for the facility. Most notably, Dr. Frederick's efforts in creating an adaptive career development program have garnered recognition within the Department of Corrections, and respect among both corrections staff and inmates. How will his role as supervisor in the interrogation of the above inmate affect his parallel roles as clinician and organizational consultant? What are the ethical considerations that must guide his supervision of the investigative process?

Brief Commentary: The rehabilitation psychologist in this case is involved in **multiple relationships**, each of which is pertinent to his employment contract. The Ethics Code does not preclude psychologists from entering into multiple relationships as long as the boundaries among the different roles are well established and do not cause impairment, risk exploitation, or harm to those persons affected. Therefore, a discussion with the associate warden regarding the potential negative impact of the interrogation activity on the roles of program developer and policy-maker within the institution should occur. The decision to move forward with implementing the organization's request should turn on thorough investigation of role boundary establishment and avoiding the fact of or perception of **conflict of interest** in the eyes of the inmate population. If the psychologist's image as a HCP within the prison population is compromised by the supervising interrogator role, career development program development may be hampered in terms of suspicions about intentions, resulting in reduced inmate cooperation with such activities. Additionally, the role of policy-maker may be impeded if the psychologist is viewed by the prison population as an enforcer of punitive organizational activities that have a negative impact on peer inmates, independent of the purpose of the interrogation process or personal responsibility of the accused fomenter of the disturbance. If this is the case, the perception of any new policy developed by the psychologist would likely be negative, inviting push-back regarding implementation.

Provided that the rehabilitation psychologist and associate warden decide on a constructive rationale for the psychologist to be involved with the inmate interrogation (e.g., arbiter, objective referee, etc.), there should be no compelling reason for the psychologist to recuse himself from this activity.

RELEVANT STANDARDS

3.04 Avoiding Harm
3.05 Multiple Relationships
3.06 Conflict of Interest
3.07 Third-Party Requests for Services
3.09 Cooperation with Other Professionals

CASE EXAMPLE 2.2

"Magical Thinking: Hope at all costs"

I. Quick Reference

Critical Incident

Utilizing the Ethics Code in the course of developing professional practice routines may lead the rehabilitation psychologist to serve as an active consultant to the rehabilitation team on matters of bioethics that cut across disciplinary lines. This second case illustrates such a role when a speech-language pathologist (SLP), Judy Montrose, seeks the counsel of a rehabilitation psychologist, Dr. Yuri Petrov, regarding ethical concerns only indirectly connected with the psychologist's practice. The issue at hand is a patient, Fred Kleem, seeking cognitive rehabilitation treatment continuation, despite lack of performance data substantiating continued improvement. The patient's perspective involves loss of hope for recovery once treatment is discontinued. Additionally, the SLP believes the patient is being prescribed treatment not justified by performance-based outcome data, perhaps for organizational financial gain. The rehabilitation psychologist is familiar with the patient because he had provided inpatient and outpatient services a year earlier and was to conduct a follow-up neuropsychological evaluation.

TABLE 2.2
CASE ANALYSIS SUMMARY

Ethical Principles	Relevant Standards	Context & Key Stakeholders	Organizational & Legal Concepts	Alternative Resolutions
I. Primary Beneficence and Non-maleficence - The RP and SLP collaborate to avoid financial and emotional harm to the patient; they simultaneously act to preserve the safety of the patient's wife	1.03 Need to clarify organization's position regarding continued billing if treatment gains cannot be demonstrated. 3.04 Avoiding harm stemming from emotional distress at possible termination—abandonment; including financial problems with out-of-pocket payment burden	- Pt. sustained a moderate TBI, completed inpatient rehabilitation program; is currently coming to the end of an OP rehab treatment course with SLP but desires continued service - The patient's wife is primary caregiver whose safety was in jeopardy early in the recovery course; is now in a position to support treatment termination and transition to other services	- Federal regulations in place regarding billing for services without substantial objective evidence of treatment gains - This regulatory control may be bypassed in this case with out-of-pocket payment, but there are organizational policies that address financial burden and payment alternatives	A. RP chooses not to advise and refers to another psychologist B. RP advises SLP to terminate therapy with rationale C. RP and SLP recommend termination to HC organization; meet with family
II. Secondary Fidelity and Responsibility - Both HCPs must present the patient's current status accurately, in order for the patient to comprehend the treatment termination planned	4.05 Disclosure regarding the limits of treatment and the natural healing course after TBI 9.03 (b) Informed consent in NP assessment required to allow the patient to make an informed choice regarding use of data for treatment continuation decision 9.10 Explaining results in understandable language 10.10 Termination of treatment needs to have an explicit rationale, along with supportive services available for the transition	- The RP who is in the position of treating the patient (testing) and recommending a supportive treatment transition strategy to his colleague - The SLP is faced with transitioning her patient in the absence of treatment data supporting continuing treatment - Rehab Center is continuing to bill the patient for services - Family Practice continues to prescribe treatment without documented functional gains	- The FP continuing to order treatment without measurable evidence of functional gains will eventually be questioned by insurance utilization review	D. RP performs neuro-psychological assessment, yielding data on which to base advice regarding treatment E. Comparative follow-up NP testing and recommendations for treatment as indicated

Principle: Beneficence and Nonmaleficence

As you read this case, keep in mind several issues as you decide in what capacity you would get involved in this case.

- What are the ethical boundaries and considerations between colleagues?
- What are the rights of patients in expecting treatment?
- How does one balance the needs of the patient with needs of the organization?
- What is the responsibility of the psychologist regarding follow up services?

Resolutions

A. ***RP chooses not to advise and instead refers to another psychologist***
   Pro
   a) Yuri keeps clear boundary such that any follow-up neuropsychological service that Yuri provides to Fred is not entangled in organizational dynamics, benefiting relationship with patient
   b) Referral to another psychologist addresses Yuri's responsibility toward ensuring appropriate services recommended
   Con
   a) Yuri's rejection of Judy's request for assistance may compromise trust built between them, jeopardizing potential future teamwork.
   b) Because of prior relationship with family, patient and spouse may feel abandoned at time of emotional need

B. ***RP advises SLP to terminate therapy with rationale***
   Pro
   a) Therapy termination is justified based on lack of progress in meeting treatment goals
   b) Rationale provides context for patient and spouse rather than outright rejection left to conjecture
   c) Yuri is viewed as responsive to collegial need
   d) SLP services can be directed toward other patients in need
   Con
   a) Emotional needs of family are not adequately addressed
   b) Ethical issues with SLP state board not adequately addressed; possible position of jeopardy for clinician given documented treatment without progress up to termination point
   c) Failure to make recommendations regarding professional relationships, as Judy also needs to close loop with family practitioner; complaints

are likely from patient to referring physician; limited communication between clinician and referral source has occurred

d) Failure to appropriately address neuropsychology service follow-up

C. **RP and SLP recommend termination to health care organization; meet with family**

Pro

a) Recognize potential risk to hospital and follow through with appropriate communication
b) Collegial support for clinician in meeting with patient and spouse to inform and support during treatment termination discussion
c) Provide collegial support in addressing policy issues and in addressing the potential ethical issue with the health care organization

Con

a) Therapy termination occurs, leaving emotional needs of the patient unattended
b) Opens the clinician to possible organizational censure for policy violation
c) Failure to recontact the family practitioner, who is therefore not prepared to respond to patient at their next visit
d) Possible referral source dissatisfaction per patient complaint

D. **RP performs follow-up neuropsychological testing on which to base advice regarding treatment**

Pro

a) Serial neuropsychological assessment can document functional change across time; provides data in support of treatment provided to date
b) Decision to discontinue treatment is data-based via external criterion; reduces risk of possible clinician decisional bias
c) Yuri fulfills previously committed professional responsibility to follow up with Fred regarding cognitive function

Con

a) Organization not informed of the decision to terminate, or the potential ethical concern
b) Opportunity to address policy issues lost
c) Possible referral source dissatisfaction, if communication lacking
d) Possible dissatisfaction by the SLP regarding emotional support

E. **Comparative follow-up testing and recommendations; with treatment as indicated—Preferred**

Principle: Beneficence and Nonmaleficence

Pro
a) *Neuropsychological assessment documentation of functional change across time; validation of treatment to date*
b) *Whether to discontinue treatment is data-based via an external criterion, and is further intended to preserve the patient's personal financial resources*
c) *Organizational policy issue addressed, with data in support of the decision-making process; possible modification*
d) *Referral source presented with data-based decision; can then be compared with the patient's perspective if a complaint is lodged*
e) *Support from a colleague in wading through the charged relationships*

Con
a) *Patient/wife distress regarding treatment discontinuation can be expected*
b) *If neuropsychological evaluation supports continued SLP services and Judy disagrees, could create threat to professional relationship*

II. Contextual Influence

Judy Montrose, an SLP employed by the rehabilitation hospital, sought consultation from Dr. Yuri Petrov, the rehabilitation psychologist who worked on the inpatient service. Judy had worked closely with Yuri for almost 10 years until she was assigned to the outpatient rehabilitation clinic almost a year earlier. The psychologist had established a reputation as an effective problem-solving consultant to professional members of the various rehabilitation teams in the organization, and Judy had successfully applied Yuri's counsel in the past. She described the patient, Fred Kleem, providing details about his course of treatment, the functional gains that had been made, functional levels yet to be achieved, and the treatment plateau that had been reached. Dr. Petrov was surprised to learn that the patient was still in outpatient cognitive rehabilitation treatment, after having been discharged from inpatient rehabilitation many months earlier. He surmised that the difficulty he had recently experienced scheduling Mr. Kleem for posttreatment neuropsychological evaluation was related to patient unwillingness to acknowledge that this outpatient treatment episode had come to an end.

Judy Montrose added that the patient had depleted his savings, had taken out a second mortgage, and was on the brink of bankruptcy from paying out-of-pocket for twice-per-week treatment; treatment that hadn't produced objectively measurable gains for almost 2 months. She had explained the conundrum to Dr. Gray, the patient's family practitioner, who had nevertheless repeatedly written prescriptions for treatment, despite lack of supporting data. Judy had also spoken to hospital management about unilaterally discontinuing treatment to avoid the patient experiencing financial ruin, but had not yet received a concrete response.

Further contextual information regarding medical history is warranted at this juncture. Because the psychologist had provided services to Fred, some of this information can be gleaned from what the psychologist knew, presented below.

Fred Kleem, a 37-year-old male, had been airlifted to St. Michael's Medical Center (Level I Trauma Center) after a crash at a masters-level motocross competition. He had sustained multiple orthopedic fractures along with an acquired brain injury (bilateral petechial hemorrhages, subcortical right frontal lobe hemorrhage; initial Glasgow Coma Scale (GCS) of 5 rising to 8 at the ER). He was hospitalized in acute care for almost 3 weeks, including 4 days in a comatose state, prior to transfer to St. Michael's Rehabilitation Center (an inpatient unit nested within the medical center).

As Fred's level of awareness improved, he began to respond inconsistently to basic functional commands. The quality of Fred's responses was serially documented as part of Dr. Petrov's acute hospital consultation. Those data figured prominently in framing the decision for rehabilitation transfer.

Fred Kleem's emergence from coma was characterized by agitation. On his admission day in inpatient rehabilitation, Fred repeatedly ripped off his hospital gown and was frequently heard screaming in pain. The latter occurred when he was touched in any manner. Risperidone had been administered for a brief period of time in response to this agitated neurologic state, along with behavioral strategies to minimize environmental overstimulation—both with moderate success. With time, the intensity of Fred's agitation had diminished. However, until Fred fully emerged from his agitated state 1 week later, he preferred to be naked. Needless to say, his rehabilitation program initially took place in his room, rather than the social milieu of the treatment gym.

With discharge home 2 weeks away, Dr. Petrov had performed a functional capacities-oriented neuropsychological evaluation to assist with outpatient treatment planning. He had hoped to meet with Fred and his wife Wilma for test results feedback in preparation for the transition home. During Fred's rehabilitation admission, Wilma had served as his primary rehab caregiver, refusing to leave the rehab center except to sleep. However, as Fred's confusion cleared, his interactions with Wilma had begun to border on abusive, triggering repeated protective staff interventions. After 2 days of this behavior, which was interfering with completion of rehabilitation tasks, Wilma was supportively asked to avoid visiting until Fred had more time to adapt to the rehabilitation setting. She was scheduled to return several weeks later to finish daily caregiver teaching prior to discharge. Wilma had accepted her role as primary caregiver in a spirit of dogged persistence, reflecting her traditional value of marital duty. However, she was also disappointed in the team for failing to correct Fred's unacceptable behavior. Fear was the most parsimonious description of her feelings toward Fred. He had episodically threatened both her personal safety and self-esteem during his periods of agitation. Wilma concluded that Fred simply wasn't the person she had married.

During the test feedback meeting, it became evident to the rehabilitation psychologist that the conflict between the patient and his wife during the inpatient rehabilitation admission was likely to continue at home. Lacking insight into his cognitive impairment, the patient found Wilma to be a convenient target for his ire when she offered corrective feedback in response to targeted problem behavior. Fred's insistence that "family business" was no one else's affair prompted Dr. Petrov to schedule several more family interventions prior to inpatient discharge. The goal of these treatment sessions was to secure a behavioral contract with Fred to protect the safety of his wife. Some progress was made during these treatment sessions to the point that return home occurred with reasonable safety precautions in place. However, Fred rebuffed, in no uncertain terms, an offer for individual outpatient treatment sessions. Dr. Petrov had also planned to work with Wilma throughout Fred's outpatient treatment course, but Wilma did not feel free to pursue treatment with Dr. Petrov if Fred wasn't involved with or accepting of intervention.

Speech-language pathology services had started twice per week after discharge, services Judy Montrose provided. Initially Fred made significant progress in both language and cognition. After about 8 additional months of treatment, however, Fred's objectively measurable progress had begun to plateau. Judy had decided to continue treatment because the patient was highly invested in the therapy, and he indicated it was helping him communicate more effectively with his wife; however, Wilma had not been present for those sessions to confirm Fred's claim. Based on this information, Judy had also worried about causing the patient emotional harm if treatment was terminated. After another month of no further improvement, Judy decided to seek the counsel of her colleague, Dr. Petrov.

Commentary

A fairly typical challenge in outpatient rehabilitation treatment is arriving at the point where a patient has maximized the utility of a physical therapy, occupational therapy and/or speech therapy treatment course and is ready for discharge from the rehabilitation therapist's perspective. However, the patient is often not emotionally ready for such a transition, especially if the condition for which treatment was rendered has not resolved… as is the case in many chronic conditions. In such cases, the patient and family may interpret the termination of rehabilitation treatment as tantamount to giving up hope for further recovery. The Ethics Code (Standard 10.10) for psychologists is not quite as clear as it appears on the surface regarding this type of situation: "terminate treatment when it becomes reasonably clear that the client/patient no longer needs the service, is not likely to benefit, or is being harmed by continued intervention." Applied to rehabilitation treatment, the standard contextually applies if one considers that objectively measurable treatment gains are lacking. The Ethics Code for SLPs also has room for interpretation. "Individuals shall evaluate the effectiveness of services rendered and of products dispensed, and they shall provide services or dispense products only when benefit can reasonably be expected" (American Speech-Language Hearing Association, 2012). The rehabilitation psychologist in this case was justified in offering further adjustment-related treatment to the patient during this emotion laden time of transition and in developing an appropriate termination plan.

If one interprets this case from the rehabilitation psychologist's perspective, the SLP believes the patient is not benefiting, and the financial loss represents a significant harm to the family. However, the patient believes that he needs the service and the family practitioner believes any perceived effort to treat helps the family cope. How much do patients' wishes drive this discussion?

Although patient and family wishes are paramount in informed consent to service, they weigh significantly less when the provider delivering the service determines that the service is no longer warranted. That said, psychologists have a responsibility to determine both benefits and harms. Honoring the patient's and/or family's wishes to continue treatment cannot be justified within the goal achievement treatment model. On the other hand, discontinuing treatment can be an emotionally traumatic experience that rehabilitation therapists as well as community health care providers are reluctant to trigger. Psychologists must be prepared to address these issues as part of the coping process with treatment decisions, including termination.

The concept of harm can vary depending on the stakeholder. In this case, the concept of just versus unjust harm comes into play in evaluating organizational aspects. Just harm could result from the decision to terminate services by essentially reducing a revenue opportunity for the organization. Just harm is akin to short-term loss for long-term gain or weighing the relative risks and consequences of different harms, where supporting nonmaleficence is the long-term benefit. In this case, a family losing their life's savings to an organization whose interventions produce no observable results is clearly an undesirable outcome. Psychologist members of APA are necessarily ethically obligated to avoid unjust harm, but may find that—in specific circumstances—just harm is an alternative worth considering.

Finally, this case highlights the importance of the components of the ethical decision-making model, particularly the psychosocial and contextual factors and stakeholders involved. Consider these changes to the case scenario: Assume that progress, although somewhat minimal, represented hope to the patient and his wife and that having this hope was fundamental to their successful coping. Similarly, assume that the SLP was reactive to the patient's abusive behavior because she had been abused in an earlier personal relationship. Therefore, her objective ability to evaluate the need for SLP services would have been compromised. While these changes do not create an ethical dilemma, they point to the need for appropriate ethical behavior to address these issues. An appropriate path of involvement could include reevaluating the patient and his wife to lay out a plan to address coping needs and to confront the SLP as a team member involved in a potentially harmful relationship with the patient. Ethical behavior demands action that can interface with multiple stakeholders with different ethical requirements, but the psychologist is clearly obligated to maintain appropriate relationships with other team members by taking reasonable steps to ensure patient safety and welfare. This is articulated in Ethical Standard 3.09 highlighting the need to work cooperatively to effectively serve the patient.

Disposition

The rehabilitation psychologist, with much patient encouragement, completed a follow-up neuropsychological evaluation to provide a richer picture of the patient's cognitive functioning. Evidence obtained during the evaluation suggested that Fred Kleem had remained impulsive in responding. He had significant wide-ranging problems with recall of both verbal and visual information, and with visual organization in particular. Although Dr. Petrov concurred with Judy's recommendation to terminate SLP services, he believed Fred could benefit from follow up occupational therapy (OT) to help with adaptive activity planning and implementation at home. This recommendation and follow-up intervention from

OT proved beneficial. Fred was able to engage in independent performance of routine chores, rather than relying on Wilma for assistance. In addition, an increase in confidence secondary to improved self-reliance helped lessen Fred's feelings of loss of control in his marriage. Short-term couple's intervention with Dr. Petrov (which was encouraged by OT, and to which Fred reluctantly agreed) also helped Fred and Wilma cope with the changes in their relationship. The treatment sessions also focused on the perception of abandonment regarding SLP treatment, which had significantly lessened when they discovered that an OT would be coming to their home.

Learning Opportunities

1. Discuss proper use and potential misuse of psychological assessment data in rehabilitation treatment planning.
2. Discuss the validity of a role for a rehabilitation psychologist in mediating ethical conflicts in rehabilitation venues, via grounding in the discipline-specific APA Ethics Code.
3. Consider under what circumstances it would be inappropriate for a rehabilitation psychologist to consult with another provider (e.g., think about multiple relationships and competence to practice).

Brief Scenario: A board certified rehabilitation psychologist, Dr. Bethany Farquhar, has been asked to communicate dire cancer prognoses to several patients by their attending physician. Dr. Millar, the attending physician, as Bethany subsequently learned from the nursing staff, is generally uncomfortable giving bad news to his patients. He considers the rehabilitation psychologist the "perfect answer" to this communication conundrum and wants her to regularly consult to his service. In response to this invitation, Dr. Farquhar has agreed (with some official encouragement, as indicated below) to be a clinical consultant to the inpatient cancer rehabilitation program. Her primary practice (employee contract) is part of an outpatient rehabilitation clinic treatment team nested within the same community health center as the cancer rehabilitation program.

Dr. Farquhar is a new hire to the health center, having completed her residency in rehabilitation psychology 7 years earlier. She most recently attained ABPP/RP diplomate status, having trained and worked in inpatient rehabilitation programs during her young career. However, she has had no previous training or experience working with individuals with cancer, much less patients deemed terminal. Her decision to take on the cancer rehabilitation consultancy was prompted by a request for a "favor" from the chief of medical staff, whom she had impressed during an interview for her outpatient position. Indeed, her psychologist position in the outpatient clinic was a first for the health center—a situation that warranted vetting her application at the highest levels. Dr. Farquhar's performance success in that role could potentially open the door for additional positions in the future. The cancer rehabilitation program was also a new venture for the growth-oriented health care organization, with major impetus for its development coming from the attending physician.

Brief Commentary: Given the weighty political responsibility that the rehabilitation psychologist shoulders in this case—breaking new ground for psychologist hires in the future—the desire to please the organizational power structure and to perform well within her broadening job description are strong motivational factors. However, the primary ethics concept pertinent to this case is **competency**; a concept that warrants a cautious approach to considering those job responsibilities. The rehabilitation psychologist has been asked and has agreed to take on a consultancy in a health care domain in which she has neither trained nor had practice experience. The Ethics Code allows psychologists to provide services in areas new to them, provided that they undertake relevant study, supervision, and consultation. While one might argue that the patients requested to be seen for communication of negative prognostic information have emergent needs for such information, this scenario does not rise to the level of an emergency. Therefore, Dr. Farquhar will have several additional responsibilities to shoulder in response to taking on this consultancy. First, she must communicate her competence **boundaries and training limitations** to the attending physician of the cancer rehabilitation program. The nature of this communication should entail an agreement with the physician to obtain technical information necessary to place the cancer diagnosis in the appropriate context for each patient referred.

There may also be a delay in beginning the consultancy, secondary to the need for the rehabilitation psychologist to secure **supervision/consultation** from a psychologist competent in working with individuals with cancer. The length of time for this training/supervisory relationship will depend on how efficiently and effectively Dr. Farquhar meets a priori criteria jointly established by the two psychologists regarding independent practice as a consultant to the inpatient cancer rehabilitation program. Knowledge of the specific professional performance requirements of the consultancy will be pertinent to negotiating the supervisory experience. This timing and supervision information should be communicated to the attending physician and administration of the community health center. It would also be reasonable for

Dr. Farquhar to request administrative funds of the health care organization to pay for such expert supervision.

RELEVANT STANDARDS
2.01 (a, c, d) Boundaries of Competence
2.02 Providing Services in Emergencies

3 Principle: Fidelity and Responsibility

FIDELITY AND RESPONSIBILITY in the Ethics Code translates into building trust within professional relationships and adhering to professional, scientific, and societal responsibilities in working with rehabilitation populations. Beauchamp and Childress (2009) comment that, "Professional fidelity, or loyalty, has been traditionally conceived as giving the patient's interests priority in two respects: (1) the professional effaces self-interest in any situation that may conflict with the patient's interests, and (2) the professional favors the patient's interests over others' interests" (p. 311). Beauchamp and Childress further state that instances of divided loyalties can occur "when fidelity to patients, research participants, or clients conflicts with allegiance to colleagues, institutions, funding agencies, corporations or the state" (p. 311). Professional responsibility reinforces the relationship between the health care professional and person(s) served, placing the professional in a position of heightened vigilance regarding protecting and preserving the interests of those served. Building trust and promise-keeping further facilitate the process of creating and maintaining ethically healthy professional relationships.

That said, theoretically favoring patients' interests over others' is not an exclusive consideration in practical application of this principle. Consider the intersection among fidelity and responsibility, beneficence and nonmaleficence, and respect for people's rights and dignity in weighing issues of confidentiality and patients' rights. Clearly, there are circumstances or legal tenets favoring safety over the patient's interests (e.g., suicidal ideation) or expressed desires in situations in which others' rights come into play (e.g., homicidal ideation) and for which the consequences are irreversible. In these circumstances, the psychologist's responsibility of protection transcends the patient's narrowly defined interests. Abuse of adults with disabilities is also intolerable, but responding to this can become complicated if state law does not explicitly proscribe such abuse and the individual (if competent to make such a decision) wishes no reporting of these incidents (see Florida Statutes: FS 825.102, for example). Does the rehabilitation psychologist favor the state's interest in protecting its citizens or the rights of the patient to make an independent choice? Where does one's responsibility lie, and what is the impact of one's professional choices on trust building? This is not unlike the debate surrounding assisted suicide in persons with disabilities who are not depressed and make an informed decision to end their lives (see Kirschner, Kerkhoff, Butt, et al., 2011, for related discussion). Although responsibility is first and foremost to the patient, as Beauchamp and Childress have championed, lines can become blurry when the patient's consequential interests do not converge with the psychologist's professional assessment. The psychologist's actions could effectively eliminate the trust established, placing the two components of this principle at odds.

Building trusting relationships is also embedded in team services and supervisor-supervisee relationships. If these relationships are strained by conflict, trust can be negatively affected, either directly or indirectly influencing patient care. The dynamic and highly regulated social environment of a health care organization is characterized by hierarchically defined roles with attendant boundaries. The varied health professional roles are expected to adhere to these social conventions. Yet, these boundaries are constantly assaulted by valid, often pressing needs of health care constituents—patients, family members, colleagues, staff, administration, and the community in which the organization resides. These role boundary "assaults" are fueled by the time-tested belief that health care institutions are staffed by caring individuals, who give of themselves in service of others. If a pressing need arises within the health care environment, the health care professional is expected to suborn any personal agenda in an attempt to address that need. However, differentially valuing one constituency (e.g., patients and families, or those in positions of authority) over others will eventually result in role conflicts that diminish trust among the other members of the health care team—reciprocal trust being a foundational component of the team treatment model. At the level of the health care organization, setting aside accepted role boundaries and responsibilities (i.e., practicing outside one's role-specific privileges), even if responding to a referral for service, risks sanction. This point is illustrated in the case examples.

CASE EXAMPLE 3.1

"The 11th Hour Consultation"

I. Quick Reference

Critical Incident

Callista Coolidge, an intern beginning her first day on the Veterans Administration Medical Center (VAMC) Consultation and Liaison service, has decided to demonstrate initiative by responding to a *stat* consultation received by the psychology service. At the time, her service supervisor Dr. Marla Borough is busy elsewhere in the medical center. Callista has had some experience with performing consultations from previous internship rotations in other health settings and feels confident that she can address the urgency of the situation while awaiting the arrival of her supervisor to engage the consultation in earnest.

Unfortunately, the intern is thrust into a situation involving an uncooperative patient in conflict with his attending physician. A rather curt phone interaction with the referring physician, Dr. Glenn, leaves the intern with a sense of urgency to intervene with the patient, whose discharge from the institution is imminent. However, upon meeting the patient, Mr. Lee, and his daughters, it becomes patently clear that there will likely be no opportunity for effective intervention.

Adding to the series of unfortunate circumstances, there is an information disconnect among the expectations of the referring physician regarding the role of predoctoral psychology interns, the limitations inherent in that position within the training structure of the VAMC, the profession's internship training and supervision requirements, and the trainee performance requirements of her supervisor. This disconnect has the intern trapped in a vortex of unknowns. She has unwittingly fallen into a trap of her own making in her desire to respond to the perceived urgency of the moment. The central issues of this case example create a push-pull effect between beneficence and responsibility, based on one's competence and appropriate professional boundaries. Imagine yourself in the role of the intern's supervisor. As you read the contextual influences, consider the following:

- What are the boundaries of service provision for trainees?
- What organizational requirements would you need to emphasize to ensure intern awareness regarding ethical decision-making?
- What factors would necessitate an immediate consultation response if you were unavailable, and what information would you provide the intern in this regard?
- What are the intern's responsibilities regarding introducing herself to other team members, and in maintaining a proper professional role within the team structure?

TABLE 3.1
CASE ANALYSIS SUMMARY

Ethical Principles	Relevant Standards	Context & Key Stakeholders	Organizational & Legal Concepts	Alternative Solutions
I. Primary Fidelity and Responsibility - Intern initiates consult without direction from her supervisor; intern fails to correct impression that she is an independent practitioner; decision jeopardizes trust with others through failure to clarify role - Intern's behavior does not characterize intern-supervisor relationship, especially early in a rotation in an unfamiliar clinical setting - Intern failed to adequately inform patient and family members that she was a supervised trainee II. Secondary Beneficence and Nonmaleficence - Risk of harm to patient, but minimized by circumstances of the incident; risk of harm to interdisciplinary professional relationships Respect for Patient's Rights - right of the patient to make independent decisions	2.01 Boundaries of Competence - Intern took initiative beyond her role as a new intern 2.05 Delegation of Work - RP supervisor needs to be explicit in her description of the intern's role on her service 3.07 Third-party Requests for Service - RP and MD need to be clear about the role of trainees on the consultation service; and the intern needs to be clear in describing her role to referral sources 3.09 Cooperation with Other Professionals - The MD and RP must mutually understand the role limitations regarding intern training as different from medical interns	- Patient—Expressing his desire to refuse treatment but his capacity to make this decision initially is unclear - Pt's daughters—in agreement with the health care team regarding smoking cessation; admit they've not successfully influenced patient's behavior - Intern—overstepped her intern role by initiating the consult - RP Supervisor—not sufficiently explicit in describing the role limitations of interns on her service - MD—made an emotionally biased decision regarding a patient; not clear about psychology intern's role limitations	- VAMC cites a violation of existing HR regulations regarding psychology intern role and limitations - The staff RP is professionally responsible for the behavior of trainees under her direct supervision; personnel action is possible - A capacitated patient has a legal right to treatment refusal - While federal statutes dealing with potential abuse of individuals with disability are typically handled under the Civil Rights Act, state statutes, with some variability, address defining and specifying sanctions regarding abuse of individuals with disabilities	A. Discipline the intern for exceeding role limitations B. Provide the intern adequate orientation regarding role boundaries along with disciplinary action C. Provide the intern adequate orientation; no intern disciplinary action given no treatment rendered, lack of patient harm and shared responsibility with supervisor D. RP counseled in HR regarding supervisory safeguards per policy; corrective action plan initiated with intern; set goal for optimal consult service performance by the end of the rotation

- What is your responsibility, compared with that of the intern, in following up with other team members after this incident?
- Should the intern be disciplined? Why or why not?

Resolutions

A. ***Discipline the intern for exceeding role limitations***

      Pro
   a) *Intern, via disciplinary action, learns the importance of operating within role boundaries; potentially reinforces previous education regarding practice boundaries and competency*
   b) *Existing policy regarding trainee role boundaries reinforced*

      Con
   a) *Motivation/intent of intern not adequately accounted for with policy-driven disciplinary action*
   b) *Lack of clarity with role boundaries suggests "casual" orientation of interns; supervisor explicit instructions lacking in this regard*
   c) *Relationship among physician, supervisor, and psychology trainees not addressed*

B. ***Provide adequate orientation along with disciplinary action***

      Pro
   a) *Intern, via disciplinary action, learns about role boundaries; bolstered by policy*
   b) *Receives proper trainee orientation; limited acknowledgment of situational motivation for trainee's actions*

      Con
   a) *Lack of acknowledgment of contextual factors and unclear whether these affected disciplinary outcome*
   b) *Communication with referring physician to correct misconception not considered*
   c) *RP unaware of, or overlooked policy regarding trainee role boundaries*
   d) *Unclear whether orientation includes introduction to other team members*

C. ***Provide adequate orientation without disciplinary action***

      Pro
   a) *Intern receives proper orientation post hoc; opportunity to explain motivation to act*
   b) *No disciplinary action given situational influence and lack of proper orientation (i.e., contextual factors taken into account)*

c) *Timing of judgmental error early in new rotation taken into account*
   d) *Educational rather than punitive model of training supported*

   Con

   a) *Responsibility for clinical action and orientation problems not assigned to either RP or trainee*
   b) *Policy ignored or ill understood regarding trainee role boundaries*
   c) *No treatment having been rendered does not change the action of overstepping role boundaries; patient refused treatment, rather than treatment being withheld or delayed pending supervisor arrival*
   d) *No recognition of potential damage to relationships with other providers*

D. **Provide adequate orientation, devise correction action for proper response to consultations, set goals regarding proper consult performance—Preferred**

   Pro

   a) *RP responsibility for lack of trainee orientation in a timely manner identified during HR (Human Resources) counseling*
   b) *Policy made known to supervisor for future implementation during trainee orientation*
   c) *Corrective action plan for trainee provides opportunity to discuss situation, personal motivation, and role boundaries*
   d) *Goals set within policy limits and supervisor expectations clarify clinical competencies to be developed by trainee throughout the practicum rotation*

   Con

   a) *Severity of HR counseling response and personnel record documentation may negatively affect RP's career mobility within the organization*
   b) *Misperception of the referring physician not addressed by RP regarding predoctoral trainee role limitations, as contrasted with medical interns*

II. Contextual Influences

Tyrone Lee, known in the military as Gunner because of his precision marksmanship, was an 88-year-old Army Air Corps veteran of World War II. Gunner was honorably discharged after taking shrapnel to both shoulders over Germany. He qualified for service-connected disability and continuing health services from his local Veterans Administration Medical Center. Gunner had used these resources sparingly over the years until recently, when he required neck/throat surgery at the VAMC for cancer of the trachea. The surgery, performed by Dr. Rick Glenn (an ENT specialist of some local renown and a Vietnam-era veteran) was deemed successful—even though the location of the cancerous tissue necessitated a tracheostomy. Gunner had been reasonably accepting of his altered visage and the plan for follow-up radiation treatments.

After the procedure, however, Dr. Glenn had ongoing battles with Gunner regarding smoking through his stoma. Besides the immediate health risk, Gunner had severe chronic obstructive pulmonary disease (COPD) and poorly controlled diabetes. All he needed was more vasoconstriction to further compromise his health. When Dr. Glenn tried to discuss smoking cessation strategies with Gunner, his patient simply produced a lopsided grin and said, "You ain't no longer giving the orders, Capt'n. I'm fixin' to call my daughters and retreat to the safety and freedom of home." After a series of similar interactions over the course of the previous few days, the frustrated physician finally gave up and decided to discharge Gunner from his service. His documentation described Gunner as an uncooperative patient who chose to ignore medical advice despite obvious health risks. As an afterthought, Dr. Glenn sent a *stat* consult (typed in CAPS in the electronic health record) to the rehabilitation psychology service (the Cancer Unit's behavioral consulting resource), asking for an immediate intervention with the patient and family around smoking cessation. He wanted this issue addressed before Gunner left the hospital. Dr. Glenn was unwilling to change the discharge time to accommodate this treatment order, as he was confident that his experienced psychology consultant, Dr. Marla Borough, could reasonably handle this pressured situation.

Callista Coolidge was a psychology intern assigned to Dr. Borough's Consultation/Liaison Service. She had just finished a health psychology rotation in the neighboring university health center, where her supervisors had rated her basic clinical skills as excellent. It was Callista's first day on the new service and her first VAMC rotation. When the consult arrived, Dr. Borough was completing a cognitive screen feedback session on the Neurology Unit, leaving Callista to await her return, reading service orientation material regarding VAMC operational regulations.

Eyeing Dr. Borough's computer screen with the STAT order icon blinking insistently, the intern decided to review and field the consultation—leaving her supervisor a handwritten note to that effect. Callista's intention was to gather contextual information about the referral question and then await Dr. Borough's arrival to discuss treatment planning. When she arrived on the Cancer Unit and had begun electronic health record (EHR) review, she realized that the patient was to be discharged within the hour. She immediately paged Dr. Glenn to discuss the case. However, his brief, dismissive interaction with Callista simply communicated his expectation that the consult be completed before the patient left the hospital.

Feeling that time was of the essence, Callista decided to make initial patient contact, hoping that Dr. Borough was not far behind. In her initial assessment of the case, Callista believed this kind of consult was right up her alley. She had spent a year working on a clinical trial involving behavioral versus pharmaceutical smoking cessation comparison. She had been well-versed in behavioral smoking cessation interventions and was confident that she could successfully begin the treatment process with the patient. Of course, Mr. Lee would have to follow up as an outpatient to complete the therapy.

When Callista entered Gunner's room, she discovered his two daughters destroying a pack of cigarettes. They had found the offending 20-unit nicotine delivery system hidden among their father's belongings that they had been packing in a suitcase. Mr. Lee grabbed an errant cigarette that had escaped the tearing and rending process, when he looked up and noticed the newcomer. Intently locking his eyes on the newcomer's uncertain face for a few moments, as if assessing the potential threat she may pose to his escape plans, he shrugged when in her hesitancy she appeared rather innocent. Gunner then turned his attention toward his daughters and their frenetic packing ritual.

Feeling acutely uncomfortable, Callista briefly tried to explain that she was a psychology intern working with Dr. Borough. She was effectively ignored by everyone in the room as the hurried process of packing was the priority. Callista then went headlong into the reason for her visit—Dr. Glenn's consult for smoking cessation. Cutting her off mid-sentence, Gunner Lee told the intern in graphic terms that he had no plans to quit smoking, emphasizing that he had a right to indulge in whatever bad habits he had a notion to enjoy. Before Callista could respond, the two daughters asserted that their father would be toeing the line on smoking, since he would be living with them in their shared apartment.

Then, like a well-oiled clockwork mechanism, the two sisters turned as a unit and finished packing Gunner's bags. One grabbed the sole surviving as-yet-unlit cigarette from her father's tobacco browned fingers and flung it in the trash. That accomplished, the daughters hustled him out of bed and into his wheelchair. They gathered his belongings and pushed Gunner past Callista toward the door. His smiling face was the epitome of satisfaction at having won a skirmish against the system. As Callista followed the procession with her eyes, she spotted a dark figure standing, partially obscured in a doorway. Dr. Borough had arrived.

Commentary

In this case, the intern's positive intentions to be professionally responsible and help the patient in the absence of the supervisor were unfortunately misguided. The intern believed that she was contributing to appropriate care by responding to a consult deemed urgent. However, incomplete consideration was given to the potential implications of responding to a consult without authorization, particularly as these consequences shape future professional relationships and may challenge currently developed skills. The intern made a judgment misstep in seeking to respond to a consult without the appropriate training in this treatment environment and without supervision. In essence, the trainee overstepped her bounds of competence and violated policy regarding supervision. The intentions of a Good Samaritan do not hold in nonemergency care in which the intern could have exercised other options (e.g., contacting her supervisor, declaring role limitations to the MD prior to consult initiation). That said, the intentions of the intern (i.e., initiate consultation to be responsive given impending discharge; hand over to Dr. Borough upon arrival) and their timing (early in the rotation) do tend to mitigate the likelihood of a specific resolution being implemented. There was no malice of intent, and the intern was naïve to the protocol. It is not unexpected that an intern would misjudge or overestimate her skill level given the combination of her previous related smoking cessation research experience and the fact that she had not yet developed any grounding in the complex VA environment, despite having some experience in the general health care system. The supervisor bears responsibility for the intern's service orientation, which should have included the specific operations of the consult service and under what circumstances, if any, the intern could make autonomous decisions to engage in patient assessment, intervention, or consultation. Goodyear and Rodolfa (2012) suggest that supervisors "equip themselves with a map that will enable them to anticipate the pitfalls leading to substandard supervision and the paths that lead to the highest levels of supervisory practices" (p. 261).

The fact that the patient was in no way harmed by the intern's role confusion does moderate some of the ethical concerns in this case, if one considers that the ultimate goal of supervision is to promote patient welfare and protect patient safety. In this case, no treatment had been rendered prior to hospital discharge. Risk of harm was further reduced by the rehabilitation psychologist subsequently offering outpatient intervention to the Lee family. It is important to note that a patient's adequately informed right to refuse treatment, even in the face of increasing personal risk of possible harm, remains inviolate. Noncompliance with health treatment recommendations can open the door for an individual being released from a treatment relationship (e.g., AMA discharge, dropping a patient from treatment, etc.). While this negative approach to securing compliance can be construed as a contingency-based incentive to "do the right thing" by complying with treatment recommendations, it remains a worrisome strategy by possibly restricting broader treatment access as a consequence of a specific treatment refusal, increasing health risk to the patient.

Disposition

Tyrone "Gunner" Lee returned to the home shared by his daughters, determined to continue smoking—a habit that began when he was 8 years old. His two concerned daughters attempted to persuade Gunner to stop smoking by establishing a house rule that prohibited tobacco use on the premises. In response to this dictum, Gunner simply moved his smoking behavior to the sidewalk in front of their property—rain or shine. Six months after returning home, a recurrence of his cancer prompted Gunner to check into Hospice, where he died peacefully with the support of palliative care.

Dr. Borough had arranged to meet on an outpatient basis with the daughters after Gunner was discharged from the VAMC. An invitation for Gunner to join this family treatment effort was not-so-politely rejected. Nonetheless, his daughters agreed to participate without him. Callista Coolidge participated in these sessions in a supervised cotherapist role—having explicitly described her trainee role to the sisters. The purpose of these family therapy sessions was to support their efforts to assist their father through his illness. When Gunner's health took a turn for the worse, the sisters benefited from this therapeutic relationship in terms of their coping with parental illness, which they viewed in part as a result of their father's choices, and eventually, loss.

Learning Opportunities

1. Evaluate your own organization's student orientation and remediation training policies and procedures. What changes do you recommend? As part of this evaluation process, make a list of content items you would include in a trainee's orientation packet. Keep in mind situations like the one above that you would want to avoid.
2. Describe an ethics competency training and evaluation approach that would address the boundary problems highlighted in this case. Design this competency approach at graduate student, intern, and resident levels of training—increasing levels of training sophistication and expertise.

Brief Scenario: Dr. Arnold Szyminsic, a senior rehabilitation researcher in the area of emotional response to physical exercise, was approached by his lab assistant with an urgent request for a meeting from a former participant in one of his ongoing studies. According to the lab assistant, during the course of engaging in an exercise protocol and follow-up assessment of emotional status, the participant had experienced somatic symptoms that concerned him. At the time, he did not disclose this problem to the lab assistant despite the lab assistant's voiced concern regarding the young man's struggles with the exercise protocol. He reported that he needed the monetary incentive contingent upon completing his participation in the study. Following up afterward with his family practitioner, along with several consultants, the participant discovered that he had a genetically linked and untreatable condition (similar to amyotrophic lateral sclerosis—ALS) that would result in further irreversible decline in physical function across the course of his life.

During the initial meeting with Dr. Szyminsic, the health issue was revealed. Additionally, this young man was intimately involved with one of Dr. Szyminsic's graduate students and did not want his condition disclosed to her. Independently, Dr. Szyminsic was aware that his graduate student was in the throes of considering dropping out of the training program to pursue a life with her boyfriend, as she was early in a pregnancy. What issues should Dr. Szyminsic focus on during this meeting? Where do his professional responsibilities lie with respect to his research participant and his graduate student?

Brief Commentary: By happenstance, the research participant's first awareness of the effects of his medical condition was revealed during the course of the experiment in Dr. Szyminsic's lab. Additionally, the severity of this condition was likely realized as the participant pushed his physical limitations in order to complete the protocol, for which he would receive needed monetary compensation. One must ask if such **monetary inducements to participate** may actually place an individual at risk of health compromise—possibly resulting in **harm**. Could the participant have felt unintentionally **coerced** to continue participation, despite emerging physical problems, in order to receive the agreed compensation? It is the **responsibility** of the researcher to build protective mechanisms into the experimental protocol when potential risk is suspected (e.g., unilateral discontinuation of the research protocol if the lab assistant suspects problems, without compromising the compensation agreement). In this case example, the lab assistant respected the participant's wishes to continue, despite misgivings. One may also ask if the **research informed consent** process was adequate, given the participant felt that he must continue struggling in attempting to complete the protocol in order to qualify for remuneration.

The principle of **responsibility** was further tested during the meeting between the researcher and former participant. The medical condition was apparently freely divulged by the young man. However, his request for **privacy** regarding personal medical information placed the researcher in a difficult position. Independent knowledge of his graduate assistant's personal quandary regarding her relationship with the young man, and his professional responsibility toward her, in terms of personal support and concern for her **welfare**, may allow the researcher latitude in his response to the young man. Since he was aware of both sides of the personal relationship issues between the research participant and his graduate assistant, the researcher could clarify the young man's responsibilities in his relationship with his girlfriend. Exploring the reasons for the young man's privacy request was first on the exploratory agenda, along with discussion of trust as the foundation of an intimate relationship. The rehabilitation psychology researcher, amply trained in reinforcing effective coping strategies in individuals with chronic illnesses, may have encouraged the young man to divulge his health information to his girlfriend on his own terms. Indeed, the young man could have been indirectly asking for guidance in this regard. Further, exploring the consequences of the young man withholding information regarding his health condition from his girlfriend essentially deprived her of the opportunity to provide supportive input to the decision-making process regarding their relationship.

RELEVANT STANDARDS

6.04(a) Fees and Financial Arrangements
8.02 (a 7, b 4, & 5) Informed Consent to Research
8.04 (a) Client/Patient, Student, and Subordinate Research Participants
8.06 (a) Offering Inducements for Research Participation
8.08 (a & c) Debriefing

CASE EXAMPLE 3.2

"You want to see my what…?"

I. Quick Reference

Critical Incident

A regional rehabilitation center referred an inpatient with traumatic brain injury to a private practice rehabilitation psychologist and other health care providers in the patient's home community for outpatient services. Because of the distance the patient lived from the hospital's outpatient rehabilitation center, that facility was impractical for ongoing care. The community-based outpatient rehabilitation psychologist had helped coordinate the postacute services in coordination with the patient's family practitioner.

After significant time and objectively measurable gains (documented via performance and serial neuropsychological test data), the rehabilitation psychologist received a request from the inpatient facility's nurse practitioner for the raw test data. The stated intent of the inpatient rehabilitation center's request for patient information was to perform "routine" follow-up evaluative services (with the potential for recommending additional treatment), services that are seemingly duplicative of the assessment and treatment the patient had already received in his home community. The rehabilitation psychologist communicated her concerns about the patient's need (or lack thereof) for further evaluation and treatment and stipulated specific requirements for release. She then received a call from the medical director of the rehabilitation program, who suggested her reluctance to immediately release the documentation was hindering the patient's treatment course. He also mentioned that legal action was pending in the case and cited a tight time line from the attorney to procure case-relevant information.

This case highlights how one values fidelity and responsibility in one's professional work and the potential conflicts among one's personal ethics, professional standards, and obligations to work with the inpatient organization. Embedded in this case are concerns regarding professional relationships as well as clear obligations based on specific APA ethical standards regarding release of test data. Therefore, as you think about the steps you would take if you were the rehabilitation psychologist responding to the nurse practitioner's request for data, consider the following questions.

- When is it appropriate to release raw test data?
- Are there any circumstances under which you would not release raw test data to an inpatient team/other referral agent?
- How would pending legal action influence your decision to release test data?
- If raw data are released, what are reasonable steps you would need to take to protect test security?
- What is your responsibility in correcting misdirected data?
- What steps can you take to prevent a potentially negative relationship developing with a referral source?
- If you discovered that another provider knowingly ordered unnecessary testing or treatment, what are your ethical obligations to challenge this action? What steps would you take next?

Resolutions

A. **Release all data**

Pro
a) *Information communicated in a timely manner to colleagues to facilitate possible additional evaluation and treatment services*
b) *Patient-controlled release of information respected*

TABLE 3.2
CASE ANALYSIS SUMMARY

Ethical Principles	Relevant Standards	Context & Key Stakeholders	Organizational & Legal Concepts	Alternative Solutions
I. Primary Fidelity and Responsibility - Care must be taken to protect patient confidentiality and provide needed services - Responsibility to actively manage cooperation among disparate treating professionals to meet patient needs II. Secondary Respect for Patients' Rights & Dignity - The patient has multiple layers of professionals representing his interests; these professionals must adequately inform the patient about his health, services provided, and consequences of decisions made - Decisional capacity is in question, but must be clear regarding the patient's wishes	3.09 Cooperation with other professionals - All rehab HCPs are bound to and well versed in the team treatment model 6.02 Confidentiality of Records - Even with the release, protecting test data is required 9.04 Release of Test Data - Standards of practice exist, with release restricted to qualified persons/ by consent 9.11 Maintaining test security - Standards of practice exist to protect copyrighted material 10.04 Providing therapy to those served by others - Coordination of services required to avoid duplication, and undue burden on the patient	- Patient - Focus of evaluation and treatment; vulnerable to undue influence from others - RP - Obligated to protect confidentiality, prevent duplicative services, and okay NP as a credible recipient of raw test data - NP—Must follow protocol for raw test data release - Attorney-Must respect proper procedure in release of test data - Family Physician - Coordinating OP services in community - Medical Director and Rocky Bay - Must avoid duplicative services and support OP continuum of care; respect interprofessional communication regulations	- RP is tasked with cooperating in resolving any conflict between ethical and legal issues and cooperating with the attorney on behalf of her patient (Standard 1.02) - In this regard, she is obligated to negotiate with the attorney regarding his provision of a qualified psychologist to review any raw data released in the case, following the standards set for such matters (NAN, 2000) - The variability in state law makes patient's part-time, seasonal fishing employment a potential point of legal contention regarding receiving Workers' Compensation benefits	A. Release all data once signed releases are received in service of efficient care B. Release all data after establishing credibility of data recipient C. Release all data once signed releases are received in service of efficient care D. Release all data after establishing credibility of data recipient E. Release all data after vetting recipients; object to all proposed services after the patient has achieved community-based outcomes F. Release all data after vetting recipients; monitor proposed additional outpatient services in light of community-based outcomes to ensure proposed services are additive and beneficial

Con
a) *No influence over reinterpretation of raw test data by recipient without direct contact between RP and NP*
b) *No quality control over expertise of raw data recipient without credentials verification*
c) *No mention of services already delivered to reduce likelihood of service duplication*
d) *No retention of case management control within the community service group (FP, RP, PT, SLP), ceding this responsibility to rehab center staff*
e) *Superficial acknowledgment of legal case implications in transfer of raw and progress documentation data; no quality control over credentials of legal consultant reviewing data; no release from the attorney*

B. **Release after establishing recipient credibility**
Pro
a) *Control over review of raw data recipient credentials to interpret material released*
b) *Patient-controlled release of information respected*
c) *Support of legal case via case record release—patient signed*

Con
a) *No mention of possible duplicative services planned by rehab center*
b) *Potentially compromised case management control of the community-based treatment team*
c) *Superficial acknowledgment of legal case implications*

C. **Release after recipient vetting and objecting to additional services**
Pro
a) *Control over review of raw data recipient credentials*
b) *Patient-controlled release of information respected*
c) *Objections to further services based on data regarding gains optimized during community treatment*
d) *Support of legal case via signed data release*

Con
a) *Potentially compromised case management control of community-based treatment team; may allow for duplicative services delivered at rehab center*
b) *Given patient's ultimate return to the community post-treatment, any ongoing service delivery may reflect a compromised relationship between patient and community team*

c) *Rejection of possibility of additional rehab center evaluation and treatment being additive, rather than duplicative; ignoring potential advantage of rehab center service resources for the patient*
D. **Release after vetting and monitor OP services in light of goals achieved—Preferred**

Pro

a) *Control over review of raw data recipient credentials*
b) *Patient-controlled release of information respected*
c) *Further rehab center evaluation and treatment monitored by community-based treatment team to discourage duplicative services; can cooperatively assist to ensure that any additional services are relevant to the patient's community's social context*
d) *Support of the legal case via signed data release (with recipient credentials review)*

Con

a) *Allows for the possibility of duplicative services if not properly monitored (e.g., contentious relationship, geographic distance limitation, etc.)*

II. Contextual Influences

Chip Fischer, a 26-year-old part-time information systems analyst, loved living and working in the Pacific Northwest, because it allowed him time to pursue his true passion, seasonal salmon fishing. He had become quite proficient at the various jobs on a commercial fishing boat, to which he contracted for part-time work during the salmon season. The regular crew came to appreciate his increasing skill—that is, until a heavy block and tackle from the rigging came loose during rough seas, striking him on the head. Chip was airlifted to a Level II Trauma Center in Port Angeles, Washington, where he underwent an emergency craniotomy for evacuation of a rapidly expanding right subdural hematoma. He regained consciousness 3 days after his surgery, demonstrating severe left-sided sensory and motor impairments, as well as cognitive processing deficits.

Chip was eventually transferred to Rocky Bay Rehabilitation Center, an acute inpatient rehabilitation facility. Although he made slow, steady progress in both physical and cognitive arenas, at discharge Chip still required some assistance with daily living tasks. Dr. Chen Yu, the neuropsychologist consulting to the rehabilitation program, had conducted serial bedside evaluations that suggested resolving moderate cognitive impairment. He elected to defer formal testing until Chip returned for his routine outpatient follow-up visit.

Fortunately for Chip, the small inland village in which he had resided for the past several years was a tight community. As the rehabilitation center's case manager put out word for help, several families volunteered to take Chip in and provide assistance. With this community support and limited home-based PT and SLP, Chip was able to return to his own apartment within several weeks. His family practice physician, after having received progress documentation from the home health treatment team, realized that Chip's cognitive processing impairments required more focused intervention—something that should not wait for the follow-up visit to the rehabilitation center. Chip was referred to Dr. Naomi Klein, a rehabilitation psychologist in a nearby town, for evaluation and cognitive rehabilitation.

Dr. Klein performed a thorough clinical evaluation, including neuropsychological measures, and began Chip's treatment. In the spirit of her rehabilitation training, she also visited Chip's apartment with his physical therapist. They devised an aggressive self-exercise and community reintegration program that yielded measurably improved function. Then, Dr. Klein gradually involved Chip in work-related task training, increasing task complexity as mastery occurred. Formal follow-up at Rocky Bay Rehab Center was postponed in order to consolidate gains in the community-based treatment program coordinated by the family practitioner and Dr. Klein. Across the 4 months after rehabilitation hospital discharge, Chip had reacquired the skill set necessary to return to independent living and part-time work (a supervised work trial, negotiated with Chip's high tech firm employer by the community-based treatment team).

At that point, Dr. Klein performed a reevaluation to document cognitive change across time. Chip performed in the average range in most cognitive domains sampled. His scores were significantly higher than those of the initial assessment. Nonetheless, his preinjury ability was estimated to have been higher. With Chip's consent, Dr. Klein contacted his family physician, the outpatient therapists, his work trial employer, and the case manager from the rehabilitation center (who was continuing to coordinate outpatient funding authorization with Chip's insurer) and provided a comprehensive report of her assessment.

The nurse case manager in the rehabilitation center also facilitated the delayed follow-up visit with the Rocky Bay outpatient rehabilitation team. Appended to that outpatient team was Dr. Yu, the consulting neuropsychologist, who had originally deferred inpatient assessment until the outpatient follow-up visit. Clearly, Dr. Yu had not anticipated that Dr. Klein would be involved in Chip's case nor that the follow-up visit would be postponed.

One week after discharging Chip from treatment, Dr. Klein received an e-mail from the case manager, asking for copies of all reports and raw test data from both assessments. She explained that Dr. Yu preferred not to perform additional testing if those data had been recently acquired. Any further treatment he determined as possibly beneficial could be tailored to Chip's test performance during Dr. Klein's second assessment.

The next morning, the patient's attorney faxed Dr. Klein a request for copies of all medical records, including raw test data. Dr. Klein's response to both inquiries was the same. She would send reports promptly after receiving patient-signed information releases, but would only release raw test data to a qualified psychologist. Then, the following day, Dr. Klein received a phone call that sparked her concern all the more. It was from the inpatient rehabilitation facility medical director, who informed Dr. Klein that his treatment team required release of the raw test data, along with the summary report documenting Mr. Fischer's progress through treatment termination. The purpose of the detailed review was to assist in future treatment planning. The medical director assured the rehabilitation psychologist that a signed release would be faxed to her before the phone call terminated.

Dr. Klein then expressed her concerns to the physiatrist by emphasizing that their shared patient had completed his outpatient rehabilitation program, as evidenced by objective and ecologically valid evaluation data from cognitive assessment and both therapeutic and vocational observational sources. Additionally, she explained the ethical restrictions on her to ensure that the credentials of the psychologist to whom the test data would be released were valid, and that safeguards against misuse of the data were in place. Thus, personal communication between herself and Dr. Yu would be necessary before data could be released. She emphasized that such precautions were considered standard of practice. Despite objections from the medical director that such an overly cautious approach to information sharing caused delays in providing services to Mr. Fischer, Dr. Klein firmly stood her ground.

Commentary

As Standard 9.04 in the 2002 Ethics Code indicates, it is now acceptable to release test data to the patient, to someone else identified by the patient on the release form, and as required by law. (See Fisher, 2012, for a discussion of confidentiality laws.) That said, Standard 9.04 also highlights the responsibility of the psychologist to weigh the risk of harm or potential misuse of the raw data prior to making a decision to release it. In this case, the intentions of the requesting physician remain unclear, and the circumstances under which the patient provided consent are unknown. The rehabilitation psychologist would be wise to verify informed consent by the patient, particularly given the psychologist has an ongoing professional relationship with the patient, and to clarify the use of the data by the inpatient rehabilitation team.

The rehabilitation psychologist already had a reasonable plan in place for review of qualifications with the neuropsychologist. Unless legally compelled to release the data, it is prudent for the rehabilitation psychologist to await the return of the neuropsychologist. Fisher (2012) reminds us that while ethics and laws sometimes overlap, they are not the same; in addition, being legally obligated to release information is not the same as being legally permitted to release information. Even under the umbrella of a subpoena, the psychologist might still consider other more limited options for release. (See Hanson & Kerkhoff, 2011 for a brief discussion of this point.) Fisher also emphasizes the importance of using a structured approach to decision-making when ethical and legal issues are involved related to confidentiality considerations. She offers a six-step model to protect patients' confidentiality and includes a list of subcomponents within each step. These steps are: (1) prepare (e.g., decide when to limit confidentiality in your practice setting); (2) tell clients the truth (e.g., acquire consent encompassing confidentiality limits); (3) obtain informed consent before disclosure (e.g., disclose without consent only when legally mandated); (4) respond ethically to legal demands for release of information (e.g., tell client about impending disclosure); (5) avoid nonmandated disclosures (e.g., establish protective policies); and (6) talk about confidentiality (e.g., provide ethics consultation). These recommendations are consistent with our general philosophy that psychologists need to be proactive in managing ethical obligations rather than finding themselves in a situation of preventable crisis management.

That brings us to two additional points of discussion raised by the confidentiality issues in this case. The first relates to test data/interpretation and other confidential personal health information faxed to a professional office. The fax machine, manned by clerical staff, typically receives business correspondence from a wide variety of sources. This fact allows the possibility of sensitive patient information being casually inspected by nonclinical staff. The confidentiality of faxed sensitive patient information must be protected under such circumstances. This might be accomplished by designation of a "confidential clinical information only" fax machine within the facility, a machine monitored by specially trained staff. If a unique machine is not feasible, then a cover sheet clearly marked confidential and a phone call to the facility immediately prior to faxing with assurance that someone is immediately available by the machine to pick up the fax and confirmation that this retrieval, in fact, occurred.

The second issue is proactively preventing the misdirection of test data to another professional's desk. This situation points up an additional need for heightened information security in the rehabilitation facility, consistent with HIPAA regulations (1996). In this case, the demonstrated integrity of both the secretary and the medical director was the only protection against inappropriate dissemination of confidential personal health information. If the medical director had discovered misdirection of the data submitted, a corrective action plan should have been initiated to reduce risk of exposing confidential material in the future.

Disposition

Chip Fischer completed his follow-up evaluation at Rocky Bay Rehabilitation Center without fanfare or problems. Indeed, the treatment plan carried out in his rural home community had provided Chip with the necessary resources to optimize his recovery. The potential conflict between the rehabilitation psychologist and medical director was amicably resolved when the rehabilitation center's routine follow-up evaluation confirmed the functional gains made by Chip since discharge. Dr. Yu, after reviewing the serial cognitive assessment data provided by Dr. Klein, elected to forego additional testing. He determined that the data, bolstered by documented performance gains in the community, validated the findings related to improved cognitive function. To the credit of both the Rocky Bay Rehabilitation Center and the community-based treatment team, a cooperative pilot project was proposed for state funding designed to strengthen the urban-rural continuum of care for individuals with disabling conditions. The out-of-court negligence (based on product liability) settlement brought Chip Fischer a modicum of financial security to offset his redefined employment status—functioning in a position of lowered responsibility, but functioning successfully without supervision. Finally, Chip returned to his salmon fishing hobby, but in a more cautious manner—avidly fishing inland streams during the annual spawning run.

Learning Opportunities

1. Describe all of the PHI (personal health information) protections that you have built into your practice in line with HIPAA and relevant state privacy statutes. Are there any important safeguards missing from your description?
2. Consider how you, as the identified rehabilitation psychologist, would have approached the rural "rehab team" cobbled together in this case, with a goal of enlisting interdisciplinary cooperation and providing coordinated care.

Brief Scenario: Dr. Hildegard Millefiglio, a rehabilitation psychologist treating an individual with spinal cord injury (SCI), discovers during the course of treatment that her patient is related to one of her husband's management consulting business clients. While she does not open that conversation with the patient, he spontaneously discovers the connection. Having found Dr. Millefiglio's creative and probing interactions with him significantly beneficial, the patient proposes a business consultancy outside the bounds of her health care profession and their working relationship that would financially benefit his relative's company, her husband,

and herself. Further, he offers to broker the consultancy arrangement. How should Dr. Millefiglio handle this potential dual/multiple relationship challenge?

Brief Commentary: **Multiple relationship** concerns come into play if the rehabilitation psychologist seriously considers accepting the business deal offered by her patient. The issues at hand are the psychologist's requirement of objectivity, competence, and effectiveness in performing her professional responsibilities in the treatment of her patient. Should a business relationship arise among the patient, Dr Millefiglio and her husband, terminating treatment and transferring the patient to another qualified psychologist would be the recommended course of action, in order to avoid a potential **conflict of interest**.

Even if the rehabilitation psychologist decides to forego the business opportunity brokered by her patient, she must deal with the inevitable consequences of turning down a good faith offer from the patient. Feelings of rejection may impede the working treatment plan that had been created. At the very least, the rehabilitation psychologist must have a pointed conversation with her patient, explaining the potential risk inherent in his business proposal and emphasizing the **adequately informed decision-making responsibility** of the patient regarding risk to the therapeutic relationship. The point of such a conversation is to actively avoid a potentially **exploitative relationship** brought about by engaging in psychological treatment with a person involved in a parallel business relationship, where lines of influence and authority are blurred. Again, if the patient elects to remain in treatment, establishing firm boundaries protecting the therapeutic relationship between the rehabilitation psychologist and her patient is paramount and an ethical obligation. The business opportunity must be foregone.

RELEVANT STANDARDS

3.04 Avoiding Harm
3.05 (a & b) Multiple Relationships
3.06 Conflict of Interest
3.08 Exploitative Relationships
3.10 (a) Informed Consent

4 Principle: Integrity

INTEGRITY IS DEFINED in the Ethics Code (American Psychological Association [APA], 2002) as actively promoting accuracy, honesty, and truthfulness in science, teaching, and practice. Effective communication with persons served can easily be extended to promoting accurate, honest communication among members of the rehabilitation team, to graduate students whom we mentor, in classroom educational activities, and with colleagues with whom research is conducted and results are conveyed. While this principle can be realized via modeling desired behavior, we are also enjoined to advocate for honesty and accuracy in others within our field, and to extend that focus more broadly to the health care system.

While the principle of integrity typically applies to individuals, it can and should be applied to organizations with whom rehabilitation psychologists are allied. Indeed, rehabilitation psychologists may consider evaluating potential consultative or employment relationships with specific individuals, groups, and/or organizations in light of adherence to this principle in objective and measurable detail. Review of policy and procedure documents, contract language, service delivery models, and marketing practices can inform the review process.

Appropriate judgment regarding professional boundaries is a related concept intersecting with the ethical principles of integrity, professional responsibility, and nonmaleficence. Psychologists must be able to successfully judge what they can and should, and cannot and should not manage to ensure appropriate representation of skills at both the individual and organizational levels. In addition, accurate self-assessment contributes to one's ability to keep professional promises, a core component of integrity. The boundaries one sets will ultimately define the type of relationship in which the psychologist will engage with individuals, rehabilitation teams, and organizations. It is also important to keep in mind that there are inherent power imbalances in therapeutic relationships. Unless dealt with deftly, mistrust can create potentially insurmountable barriers to successful professional relationship building and maintenance.

The landscape becomes even more complicated when the psychologist is involved in multiple relationships. Setting functional boundaries across these relationships is critical to ensure promises made are kept in an ethical manner. When accuracy and honesty in communication are diminished within the complex health care environment, the effectiveness of services provided is likewise affected, sometimes leading to misperceptions and negative outcomes. Psychologists feeling pressure to perform, place themselves at risk for poor decision-making that could lead to compromised relationships or worse, inappropriate conduct jeopardizing patient welfare.

> CASE EXAMPLE 4.1
>
> "Consumer-driven health care gone bad"

I. Quick Reference

Critical Incident

The inpatient rehabilitation psychologist in this case example finds himself in a difficult situation when the boundaries among multiple roles he plays within the rehabilitation team are vaguely defined. Dr. Hammer must confront a 58-year-old patient, Angie O'Tensin, with a remote history of T7 paraplegia, and a more recent history of alcohol abuse, poor self-care, and a motor vehicle accident resulting in multitrauma injuries (but no traumatic brain injury), who refuses to be discharged—despite having met all of her discharge goals. The inpatient rehabilitation program for this patient has been stressful for everyone on the team, including the patient. However, in having to confront the patient's refusal to leave the facility, all hope of maintaining therapeutic rapport between the patient and the rehabilitation psychologist evaporated.

Angie had a recent history of idiosyncratic behavior that created conflict between her and members of her local community. Prior to the recent decline in socially appropriate behavior, she had been an effective activist on behalf of persons with disabilities. Her contrary behavior while in the rehabilitation facility was apparently an extension of her recent pattern of emotional and behavioral decline.

The rehabilitation team and administration of the organization were frustrated with Angie's position of steadfast refusal to vacate the facility after being discharged. The rehabilitation psychologist's ability to negotiate a "peaceful solution" to the escalating emotionality surrounding the situation had been diminished by the patient viewing the psychologist in the role of the rehabilitation team's tacit enforcer. Any trust that had been built early on in the admission had been eroded, as the patient evidenced determination to remain in the rehabilitation center for an undefined period of time—until she was ready to leave on her own terms.

Imagine that you are the rehabilitation psychologist—the person with whom the team has placed their hopes of resolving this matter. In order to effectively resolve this apparent stalemate and maintain appropriate integrity, think about the following issues.

- How is your role defined on this rehabilitation team?
- With what team members, if any, do you have to clarify your role?
- Would you approach the patient regarding discharge given your therapeutic relationship and, if so, how?
- What is your responsibility to the organization regarding provision of service versus discharge for this patient?
- Do you think that you can objectively evaluate your roles at this point? Why or why not?

Resolutions

A. **Engage in discharge planning; recommend patient remain in facility**

Pro

a) *Patient remains in a safe environment, with proper medical supervision and ongoing care*
b) *Avoids confrontation with patient that degrades trust and potential for future constructive facility utilization (anticipating likely future needs for rehabilitation services)*
c) *Avoids possible negative public image, if the patient pursues media exposure*
d) *Control over length of stay rests with the patient, reinforcing patient preference orientation of the organization*

Con

a) *Patient has demonstrated medical stability and modified independence with activities of daily living*
b) *Confrontation with patient may not be avoidable, if her position is not negotiable*
c) *Patient control over discharge timing ignores criterion of goal achievement, organizational policy, standards of care, and funding agency regulations*

TABLE 4.1
CASE ANALYSIS SUMMARY

Ethics Principles	Relevant Standards	Context & Key Stakeholders	Organizational & Legal Concepts	Alternative Solutions
I. Primary Integrity - The multiple roles played by the psychologist proved to be a differentiation challenge in a patient with emotional and behavioral problems; importantly, his supportive role was compromised as patient-team contention arose II. Secondary Respect Rights and Dignity - Limits with respect to honoring patient preferences are often ill-defined; in this case, the patient's manipulative character served to challenge the rehab process of incorporating patients into team decision-making Nonmaleficence— Ill-defined role boundaries place the patient at risk of harm and team relationship in jeopardy if role unfulfilled	3.04 Avoiding harm - Requirement to provide a safe discharge plan and keep the patient's welfare at forefront of decision making 3.09 Cooperation with other professionals - Complexities of team roles and communication 4.05 Disclosures - Only information pertinent to the case being shared 4.06 Consultations - Inherent in interdisciplinary rehab setting; broader application in this case (see ethics committee) 10.10 Therapy termination - Therapeutic role compromised by team communicator role; treatment impeded	Patient-team communication compromised by manipulative behavior RP - Therapeutic role compromised by role as team limit setter Rehabilitation Team - Treatment effectiveness diminished as conflict characterized the relationship with the patient Organization's Leadership - Essential conflict between treatment mission and rehab process adherence Ethics Committee - Responsibility to ensure due care provided, safety needs met	- Organization committed and obligated to provide high quality treatment and a safe discharge plan; potentially compromised by patient behavior - Patient does not have unconditional right to inpatient care so legal support may be necessary if patient refuses to leave - Legal actions considered should allow for safe transfer of patient to discharge setting; consideration of trespassing violation under state property law - Ethics Committee consult arranged to assist with safe disposition	A. Engage in discharge plan; recommend patient remain in facility in a nonparticipative role until she declared herself ready to discharge B. Engage in discharge plan; recommend discharge with public transport arranged to deliver patient to her doorstep; home health arranged for at-risk status C. Engage in discharge plan; recommend discharge via law enforcement under the trespassing charge, which ensures safe transport and assist with entry into the home and removal of the weapon; Home Health Care follow-up arranged D. Delay discharge 2 days and tell patient date; make arrangements with home health services and declare to patient as each discharge step is in place E. Do not engage in plan; define role boundary and transfer responsibility for discharge management to the social worker

    d) *Inappropriate bed utilization potentially denies another individual admission and access to needed services*
    e) *Engagement with team not apparent; discharge recommendation likely to result in negative reaction by patient*

B. **Engage discharge plan; recommend patient discharge with public transportation home and Home Health Care follow-up**

Pro

    a) *Patient discharged, assisted to the door; provided with door-to-door transportation*
    b) *Follow-up Home Health Care (HHC) assist per demonstrated need provided, with an alert for Social Services to be involved as part of the HHC team*
    c) *Respects discharge criteria (standard of care, regulations, etc.) regarding timing, destination, and follow-up care*
    d) *Plan is consistent with team's recommendations*

Con

    a) *Patient objections to "forced" discharge leads to confrontation; could bring charges of assault with transfer assist provided*
    b) *Confrontation may create patient motivation to bring negative media exposure to the facility*
    c) *Confrontation presents negative image of the facility to peer patients, whose queries in the event may not be adequately addressed because of patient privacy and confidentiality requirements*

C. **Engage discharge plan; use law enforcement to transport under trespassing charge; arrange for HHC follow-up (including Social Services)—Preferred**

Pro

    a) *Patient's legal status compromised by charge of trespassing, limiting ability to find fault with organization from legal and media perspectives*
    b) *Patient discharged; with home community police escort as witness to proper procedures provided for safe return home (including removal of weapons from the house)*
    c) *Follow-up HHC assist in the home; can alert Adult Protective Services if the patient is considered a danger to self or others*
    d) *Respects standard discharge criteria*

Con

    a) *Confrontational role of RP detracts from therapeutic role vis-à-vis team and patient, inhibiting effective treatment of patient*

b) *Potential for peer patient distress, given necessary limitations of explanatory information available (privacy)*
c) *Unfortunate legal confrontation between patient and HCO*

D. **Establish temporary delayed discharge date; follow structured steps toward discharge and announce each step achieved to the patient**

Pro

a) *Provides the patient unequivocal evidence of set discharge, with increased adjustment time, potentially reducing need for confrontation*
b) *Clearly announcing each step taken toward discharge communicates team's intent regarding impending discharge date*
c) *Potentially avoids negative backlash with the team*
d) *Balances patient's and team's interests in a controlled manner*

Con

a) *Manipulating application of discharge criteria creates a future slippery slope precedent for discharge decisions*
b) *Service to another patient is delayed*
c) *Poor coping behavior by patient is reinforced*
d) *Delay may not succeed; wasting valuable resources and creating team resentment*

E. **Do not engage discharge plan; refer to case manager**

Pro

a) *Potential opportunity to rebuilt patient's trust in the RP and team*
b) *Respected colleague with more experience in managing discharge planning takes lead*
c) *Communicates role boundary to team*

Con

a) *Imposes a role boundary inconsistent with previous actions—diminished authority*
b) *Angers team, who view this decision as abandonment*
c) *Creates inappropriate power differential within the team*
d) *Reinforces negative patient behavior (if actions interpreted as abandoning the team)*

II. Contextual Influences

"I don't care what you say, doc, I am NOT movin' from this bed." The words spat in a sharp report from Angie O'Tensin's lips like a fiery volley from the barrel of a shotgun.

Dr. Jack Hammer's therapeutic relationship with Angie toward the end of her admission could best be described as contentious—resulting in increasingly infrequent, but important contacts—by patient preference. This situation was due, in part, to the fact that the rehabilitation psychologist had actively pursued the role of "official mouthpiece" of the rehabilitation team when Angie began to push back regarding her proposed discharge timetable. He also was the one to provide reality checks to her overly negative performance self-evaluations. Dr. Hammer's discharge recommendations included outpatient alcohol abuse treatment, with an appointment arranged via her case manager. Needless to say, the patient rejected that offer of further assistance.

Angie recently sustained rib and hip fractures in an alcohol-related motor vehicle accident that had required a total hip arthroplasty (THA). Ms. O'Tensin had a 28-year history of T7 paraplegia, the result of an earlier motor vehicle accident, with subsequent rehabilitation in another state. There was a more recent history of repeated hospitalizations in several different locales following her spinal cord injury related to pressure ulcer repairs, kidney infections, several lower limb fractures (related to long bone decalcification—osteoporosis), a failed nonvoluntary admission for alcohol intoxication, and repeated bouts of pneumonia.

Angie and her then-husband Miles had settled in Parchville, a small rural community, two decades earlier. That was shortly after the onset of her spinal cord injury (SCI). She had found employment as an office manager in the village's only high tech firm, a job she had then held for more than 10 years. That job suddenly vanished when a large corporation bought the firm and moved it out of state. Angie divorced Miles when she was 46, due to irreconcilable differences revolving around her increasingly evident alcoholism. Childless and in need of a change, she gave Miles most of their shared resources (except for her adapted vehicle) and left the house. Angie then isolated herself in a dilapidated but accessible double-wide mobile home with a small menagerie of stray animals 25 miles from town. Her income was limited to meager monthly disability retirement allotments, and her infrequent health care visits reluctantly occurred in the local ER.

Finalization of her divorce proved to be a symbolic watershed event. Angie slowly began to neglect her somatic and social responsibilities associated with her long-standing, successful social activism for persons with disabilities. She became sullen and angry, alienating virtually all of her former friends and increasing her alcohol consumption. She experienced several altercations with her neighbors after damaging their properties with her car when she was intoxicated. She posted a "No Trespassing" sign and obtained a shotgun, which she was known to discharge in the air for the purpose of deterring visitors. Angie appeared to delight in social conflict, but quickly returned to sullen sedentary status when the furor died down.

The admission to Ajax Inpatient Rehabilitation Center, to which Angie had been referred by her orthopedic surgeon after the hip fracture, had been a field day for her. She successfully played rehabilitation staff against one another, threw insults at them, and had manipulated therapy attendance just enough to fall shy of mandatory discharge based on lack of progress. She had carefully honed the ability to thoroughly negate progress through inaction, just like pushing a "reset button." Employing arguments based on countering paternalistic health care decision-making that ignored her wishes and functional goals, Angie had already managed to extend her admission by almost a week.

However, the team's imposed discharge day had finally arrived. Angie's self-care and mobility skills were deemed acceptable by all objective measures, warranting her return home. Angie argued, as a veteran of disability advocacy campaigns, that she was not adequately prepared to leave. In order to stack the cards in her favor, Angie complained of continuing hip pain and refused a follow-up care plan, deeming it woefully inadequate to meet her complex needs.

As if her perceived stresses were not enough, when Angie had been hospitalized, the neighbors pleaded with the Humane Society for intervention on behalf of her abandoned animals. As a result, the menagerie had been collected and adopted out, one and all. A well-meaning rehabilitation team member had relayed this information to the patient on the day before discharge, so that she could emotionally prepare herself for the return to a dwelling devoid of animals. Angie again balked, saying that there was no way she'd return home until her "furry family" was returned intact.

Meetings between Dr. Hammer and the patient the morning of discharge had produced no workable discharge agreement. The patient-psychologist meetings were followed by serial visits from the attending physician, the risk manager, and finally the hospital administrator—all to no avail. Apparently, Angie had drawn a line in the sand—she was resolute in her determination to stay in the rehabilitation hospital, stating only that her criterion for return home had not been met—a criterion that she steadfastly refused to define. This impasse triggered an ethics committee consultation. The upshot of the committee's deliberations was to move forward with the discharge plan with Home Health Care safety monitoring included. If the patient refused again to vacate the premises, the county sheriff's office would be contacted with a trespass complaint. The committee contacted the legal department to explore patient and property rights. They then moved forward with specific recommendations for case management. Fortunately, the patient had had enough contact with local police over the years since her divorce that the case manager had no problem locating an officer familiar with her, and willing to pursue the facility's complaint.

Commentary

The tragedy in this case is the contamination of the rehabilitation psychologist's supportive/advocacy role by serving in the capacity of team spokesperson. The psychologist acted as if those two roles could not be adaptively melded. Instead, he considered them as virtually mutually exclusive. The patient found this artificial dichotomy between the two roles a convenient lever to use against the psychologist's hopes of achieving an adaptive professional relationship with her in either instance. In essence, the psychologist failed to set boundaries that would facilitate patient protection and welfare. His actions became one of "risk of harm by omission." By failing to appropriately define his responsibilities, the psychologist consequently failed to provide potentially helpful treatment to facilitate patient coping.

This may have been a circumstance under which the psychologist's personal characteristics (e.g., desire to be the spokesperson) and the situational pressures (e.g., team stress and expectations) overshadowed the emotional needs of the patient. He therefore made an error in judgment regarding the significance of his relationship with the patient as it impacted patient progress. In maintaining integrity in setting professional boundaries, psychologists need to be reasonably confident that changing roles and entering new relationships will likely provide benefit and avoid negative consequences (e.g., disrupted therapeutic relationships). In this case, had both roles been combined more effectively, the contentious nature of the patient-psychologist interactions may have been avoided, and the magnitude of team distress might have been diminished. Exploring the patient's negative emotionality surrounding the thought of returning home might have produced a more adaptive response and avoided the confrontation with legal authorities.

The reader may also benefit from a review of organizational rights, roles, and responsibilities vis-à-vis persons served, employees, and the community in which the HCO is nested in Leonard Weber's (2001) book on health care organizational ethics. It is well within the ethical purview of health care organizations to actively balance the needs of individuals with the responsibilities of organizations to protect their personnel and programs in the context of the community.

Disposition

The ethics committee's recommended plan was put into action on the scheduled discharge date. The dramatic show of resistance abruptly ceased when the patient saw the familiar face of the county sheriff's deputy who had entered the room. This deputy had actually visited Angie's home on several occasions in the past to investigate neighbor complaints. He formally introduced himself, acknowledging the previous contacts, and explained the charge of trespassing. He told Angie that he would personally escort her to her mobile home outside Parchville. Without any further outbursts, a sullen and embarrassed Angie O'Tensin received Ajax Rehab Center's first police escorted discharge.

Waiting at her home when she arrived, a duo of Adult Protective Services (APS) investigators greeted Angie. They began their assessment under the watchful eye of the deputy, who had wisely decided to remain until Angie had heard all the ramifications of the investigation. The two investigators informed her that Home Health Services would be in place the next morning, as well as mental health follow-up, teamed with enrollment in the recommended outpatient substance abuse treatment program. When the APS team had completed their first of several planned visits, they departed along with the deputy, who had requested and been given Angie's prized shotgun. Like it or not, Angie O'Tensin's life was about to change again—hopefully for the better.

Learning Opportunities

1. How would you have handled the role definition challenge with this patient had you been in Dr Hammer's position?
2. Imagine that you are Dr. Hammer's associate, observing the events surrounding this case. Develop that scenario from the perspective of yourself as an observer, and Dr. Hammer as the individual involved in the case, creating sample dialogue that might ensue.

Brief Scenario: Rodney Lightwing is performing rather poorly in your undergraduate Health Issues in Disability course. You, the professor, have noticed him sleeping in class, video gaming during lecture, being late on occasion and sitting alone, with only rare superficial interactions with the other students. He is in real danger of failing your course. You know that meeting with him is important in order to alert him to his precarious academic situation. However, in your only interaction with him early on in the semester, you had the distinct impression that Rodney was having difficulty processing your interaction. He appeared distracted and aloof, but denied any problems, and had interacted without a hint of disrespect. Now that you strongly suspect that performance problems do exist, how can you accurately and honestly communicate with your student regarding his risky academic status, and simultaneously address what appear to be cognitive, behavioral, and/or emotional problems, all within a trusting professional interaction? Generate a plan to approach this at-risk student in support of adaptive change, with active guidance from the Ethics Code.

Brief Commentary: It is important to mention at this juncture that ethics principles overlap significantly in complex social situations. Our emphasis in this example will focus on integrity, rather than responsibility—both of which apply in equal measure.

The rehabilitation psychologist professor has **dual roles** and attendant responsibilities in this case—that of educator and as an advocate and supporter of his students within the bounds of a trusting professional relationship. Integrating those roles in a manner that is **beneficial** to the student is a priority. The upcoming meeting, by reason of concerns regarding the threat to the student's academic standing (a concrete **harm**), can reflect those dual responsibilities. On the one hand, an investigation of possible reasons for the student's apparent inability to effectively engage the course materials and content could ensue. On a parallel track, clinical observation and discussion of the student's suspected cognitive processing problems regarding topic maintenance, logical sequencing, reasoning, and problem-solving could occur.

Regarding the former topic, the professor can engage in focused discussion with the student regarding strategies that may allow Rodney to catch up with the class, including crafting additional class projects that can boost his grade. The latter track may involve discovering potential etiology for the cognitive processing challenges demonstrated by the student, along with potential referral for evaluation and treatment if warranted—including introducing university student counseling and disability resources. Exercising both roles in an open and honest manner that the student can accurately process, the professor can demonstrate integrity by his efforts to interweave accurate feedback regarding academic standing, along with exploring accommodations, and simultaneously address likely disability issues. Establishing **trustworthiness** in the professor-student relationship is critical in reducing the risk of alienating this obviously distressed student.

RELEVANT STANDARDS

3.04 Avoiding Harm
3.05 (a 1) Multiple Relationships
7.03 (b) Accuracy in teaching
7.04 (2) Student Disclosure of Personal Information
7.06 (a) Assessing Student and Supervisee Performance

CASE EXAMPLE 4.2

"I can't treat my patient...."

I. Quick Reference
Critical Incident

Dr. Amie, the consulting rehabilitation psychologist to an inpatient rehabilitation program, is confronted by a colleague who interprets (with some support from her licensing board) a medical record in an overly narrow fashion. The result of this interpretation is an ethics-based refusal by Juanita Mann, the speech-language pathologist (SLP), to treat a patient poststroke because of a putative medical condition that, if valid, is refractory to cognitive rehabilitation treatment.

The patient in question, Buster Stonedancing, readily admitted that aging has affected his ability to quickly recall new information. However, he adamantly disputed the "possible dementia" statement in his medical record. He cited multiple behavioral examples of his ability to live independently in the community prior to his stroke, offering to have his neighbor and friend corroborate his story. At the same time, he demonstrated a need and desire to improve his current perceptually mediated attention impairment through cognitive rehabilitation service provision. His goal was to return home, with assistance—if required.

Having performed an assessment, the results of which challenge the isolated reference to "possible dementia" in the acute hospital medical record, the rehabilitation psychologist attempted to rectify the problem. Clearly defining his roles as service provider and program consultant to the team, he attempted to support his rehabilitation team colleague in this stressful situation, secure needed treatment for the patient, and coordinate a solution that extended beyond the bounds of the rehabilitation facility. In order to uphold the principle of integrity, the psychologist would need to accurately and honestly represent these roles, follow through on the declared roles in service to the patient, and avoid misguided decisions related to role implementation. Therefore, the following issues must be considered as you review this case.

- How can the psychologist be of help to the speech-language pathologist given his current role on the team?
- Are multiple roles either necessary or desired to serve the patient? If so, is it wise to enter into more than one role in this case?
- Can the multiple roles the psychologist plays potentially pose a risk to the patient?
- How might the psychologist's choices regarding engaging in multiple roles jeopardize or benefit the relationship with the team?

TABLE 4.2
CASE ANALYSIS SUMMARY

Ethical Principles	Relevant Standards	Context & Key Stakeholders	Organizational & Legal Concepts	Alternative Solutions
I. Integrity - the RP provides patient services in an accurate and professional manner to address his needs dictated by his condition; he advocates for service availability in accord with patient needs II. Secondary Beneficence and Nonmaleficence - The patient benefits from services provided to ameliorate the effects of his stroke; harm is avoided by provision of available services warranted by his individual health status	1.02 Conflict between ethics and legal authority - Appropriate advocacy to weigh the case on individual merits 3.09 Cooperation with Other Professionals - RP works with the MD and SLP to eliminate barriers to patient services created by initial board decision 4.05 Disclosures - The patient must be made aware of the vague dementia reference in the context of his functional skills 6.06 Accuracy in reports to funding agency - Medicare must be appraised of the unique circumstances of this case that warrant an exception 9.01-.03 Assessment - Data summary from the cognitive tests estimating the patient's functional status given his mild cognitive impairments included in the medical record 9.10 Explaining test results - Data explained in ecologically valid manner	- Patient - New stroke layered on preexisting mild cognitive impairments influence available treatment - RP - Provides needed services and advocates for withheld services - SLP - Feels ethically compelled to deny needed services - MD and Rehab Program - Advocates for proper service provision based on the patient's needs and functional level rather than a vague diagnostic reference - Neighbor - Potential caregiver; and a source of baseline patient information	- State and federal regulations are implemented per state law and practice regulations, which introduce variability in interpretation - This variability creates the possibility of allowing a variance from standard rule interpretation if a case can be made for patient benefit from that proposed treatment - Sought advice regarding Medicare regulations to assist planning	A. Take no action with SLP; comply with the initial ruling from the board and deny needed services B. Assist in providing the state board with evidence in support of an interpretive variance to allow needed treatment C. Provide the needed treatment without alerting the regulatory body, per valid patient need D. Provide collegial support but avoid getting involved in SLP board issues

Principle: Integrity | 65

Resolutions

A. ***Take no action with SLP; comply with initial board ruling***

Pro

a) *Follows advice of professional board based on chart reference, acceding to expertise/authority*

Con

a) *Denies treatment services to patient in need*
b) *Assumption of valid, evidence-supported reference in medical record—questionable approach in the face of new evidence challenging that reference*
c) *Absence of apparent investigation into details of the case by board representative before rendering an opinion; based on second-hand report*
d) *Variance from policy of HCO regarding patient care and treatment service availability*
e) *May create conflict with SLP in future based on potential emotional reactions to inaction, especially if patient's status deteriorates when treatment was available*
f) *Missed opportunity to offer professional assistance to/support professional relationship development with colleague*

B. ***Assist in providing board with evidence of needed services—Preferred***

Pro

a) *Provide extenuating evidence to state board challenging the putative statement regarding dementia; argues for variance from policy/recommendations*
b) *Provide services to patient in need*
c) *Follow facility policy regarding service provision for rehabilitation admissions*
d) *May serve to prompt board review of policy regarding service denial for specific diagnoses*

Con

a) *More formal presentation of case documentation to the board may prompt an investigation, potentially delaying needed service provision to the patient*
b) *Failure to alert HCO regarding potential ethical challenge for advice regarding treatment delivery*
c) *Risk of SLP feeling some coercion regarding decision if RP insensitive to team dynamic and/or SLP has any ambivalence regarding recommendation*

C. ***Provide needed treatment without other notification***

Pro

a) *The patient receives needed services despite concern regarding ethics violation*

Con

a) *HCP risks state board sanction of service delivery; challenge arises without notification or consultation*
b) *Facility risks criticism for allowing board policy-prohibited service delivery*
c) *Potential long-term jeopardy regarding team role if sanction occurs*
d) *Potentially place colleague at risk, damaging team relationship*

D. ***Provide collegial support but avoid board issues***

Pro

a) *Avoids entanglement with another discipline's interpretation of ethics and regulatory issues not directly related to psychological services*
b) *Recognizes importance of maintaining collegial relationship on some level*

Con

a) *Fails in responsibility to advocate for services the psychologist believes would benefit the patient*
b) *Misses opportunity to enhance collegial trust*

II. Contextual Influences

Timothy "Buster" Stonedancing, a tall, lean, elderly Native American, rarely missed an opportunity to share a joke, a political anecdote, or a simple friendly greeting. Buster's charm and wit placed all the residents in the Last Hurrah Care Center at ease. Buster had resided in the subacute rehabilitation unit for approximately 2 weeks after surviving a right hemisphere middle cerebral artery infarct, which had left him inattentive, hemiparetic, and with left visual field neglect. He had recently completed a cognitive screening with the facility's consulting rehabilitation psychologist, Otto N. Amie, PhD. Dr. Amie had found additional evidence of memory and reasoning deficits (both mild and not expected by virtue of his admitting diagnosis). However, there was a vague reference to possible "dementia of unknown etiology" in his preadmission medical record. Importantly, the severity of Buster's cognitive problems, as assessed by Dr. Amie, did not warrant a definitive diagnosis associated with a dementing process.

At Buster's initial team conference, the physical and occupational therapists shared self-care and mobility data, with the overall functional picture painted in a positive light. Dr. Amie then summarized his cognitive screening data, allowing that there was some mild cognitive impairment beyond what the team would expect from a right cortical stroke. Nursing reported that bowel and bladder functions were improving, and safety had not been a concern despite the visual field neglect. A positive trajectory for Buster's rehabilitation progress was expected. Then, Juanita Mann, the speech language pathologist interjected, stating that she was unable to treat Mr. Stonedancing because her ethics code forbade her from offering treatment for a condition that could not reasonably benefit from intervention. The team asked for clarification, and Ms. Mann stated that the mention of dementia in the medical record effectively precluded her from treating the patient. She added that a contact with her licensing board had supported a conservative interpretation of the medical record. However, she agreed to cooperate with the rehabilitation psychologist and attending physician in an effort to dispute that oblique dementia reference in the medical record, utilizing objective measurable performance data. She concurred with the team that the patient needed her interventions.

Buster was a 72-year-old stroke survivor, who had entered the Last Hurrah Care Center (and subacute rehabilitation program) outside the small town of Desolate, Montana (where the moose outnumbered the populace 5:1). In addition to impulsive, inattentive behavior and mild-moderate left visual field neglect, Buster was forgetful and had minor problems with complex reasoning. This was noted despite his college degree in agricultural science. Buster had lived independently on a portion of his ranch acreage prior to his present illness, although he had recently hired itinerant ranch hands to till his land and manage his cattle herd. His rehabilitation goal was to return home with intermittent supervision provided by his neighbor and friend, Ewell Gibson. Mr. Gibson was a widower, a retired engineer, and 12 years Buster's junior.

The first step in advocating for their patient saw the occupational therapist and rehabilitation psychologist collaborating in designing specific activity of daily living (ADL) tasks unique to Buster's measured functional cognitive status to be accomplished during an upcoming home visit. Fortunately, the completed home evaluation demonstrated that Buster could function safely within his home, with intermittent supervision and assistance from his neighbor Ewell, who willingly participated (with patient consent) in caregiver training. Driving was prohibited until Buster had followed up with his family practitioner and had completed a formal in-car driving evaluation.

Drs. Amie and Leon (the attending physician) then collaborated in generating a letter supporting continued cognitive rehabilitation treatment for their patient based on his cognitive needs. The letter emphasized a number of factors that directly impacted the clinical situation. First, the putative diagnosis of dementia in the medical record was determined to be an indirect reference to clinical observations of cognitive processing problems, without the required assessment to provide validating data. Second, current cognitive assessment data were detailed, documenting mild processing difficulty. Those data did not meet diagnostic criteria for dementia, but indicated that the patient could likely benefit from intervention. Further, the letter specified both premorbid and current learned compensations spontaneously employed by the patient to accomplish activities of daily living, necessitating only intermittent supervision. Finally, the psychologist and physician offered a collaborative expert opinion that, with further improvement demonstrated in the rehabilitation program, Buster would be able to safely return home with temporary intermittent supervision.

The speech-language pathologist concurred that the letter accurately summarized Buster's current status and demonstrated ability to acquire and utilize new functional information. She presented the letter to her state licensing board, and requested a conference call to resolve this service conflict in a timely manner. Both Drs. Amie and Leon agreed to be participants in that conversation.

In preparation for the state board conference call, Ms. Mann and Dr. Amie contacted the local Medicare office for an interpretation of the regulations. They had faxed Buster's release to share pertinent information for the sole purpose of clarifying interpretation of the regulation in his case. The representative stated that the absence of a formal dementia diagnosis gave the treating professional some latitude.

The conference call to the state board occurred the next day. The data-heavy discussion ended with an agreement for the board to consider interpretive latitude after a review of the medical record to document clinical benefit. The team requested a rendering of a timely decision, given the ongoing rehabilitation program and discharge time frame. This approach was agreeable to the board members participating in the conference call, who expressed their appreciation for the comprehensive nature of the data provided for their review. The board members added that individual case determinations were certainly within their purview, and appeared warranted in light of data provided. A decision to pursue cognitive rehabilitation treatment was returned within 48 hours.

After the ruling, Dr. Amie requested a team meeting with the purpose of closing the communications feedback loop. The team discussed the importance of individual team members consulting with their colleagues regarding making decisions that may adversely affect the quality of a patient's rehabilitation program—in this situation the potential overemphasis of the sanctioning component of the SLP's ethics code at the expense of providing practical clinical guidance on behalf of the person served.

Commentary

In this case, the psychologist's choices that involved clearly defined dual roles (i.e., service provider and consultant to the rehabilitation team) were consistent with his scope of practice. There was minimal risk to his relationship with the patient and the SLP if assistance failed to influence the outcome. Therefore, the psychologist's defined roles and associated actions appeared sound. The rehabilitation psychologist did not lock himself into a rigidly defined role structure. Instead, he considered the patient's interests and his potential indirect contributions to patient benefit. The case also illustrates that the principles of integrity, responsibility, and beneficence are intricately interconnected and that the psychologist can successfully uphold these principles when balancing different roles. By keeping his promise to serve the patient and the team, the psychologist chose actions that promoted both constructive organizational and individual relationships.

Disposition

Timothy "Buster" Stonedancing returned home after successfully completing his rehabilitation program. Ewell Gibson provided the promised supervision until Buster convinced him (through his actions) that he no longer needed to "hound dog" him. Buster lived successfully (escaping the health care system) for almost 7 years, keeping regular company with Ewell, who came to treasure Buster's pacific view of the world. Buster died peacefully while resting during a walkabout, back supported against a large rock, looking out over his beloved mountains. Ewell had accompanied Buster on that walk, somehow knowing that this would be their last together.

Learning Opportunities

1. Think of examples of organizational and/or governmental rule and regulations that have fallen short of their intended purpose, negatively influencing individuals with whom you have worked. What resolutions might apply to such challenging situations? Compare your resolutions with actual outcomes.
2. Think of a situation in which providing accurate, honest, and open professional communication could possibly result in emotional distress for an individual. With such a situation in mind, explore the issue of paternalism that influences health care decision-making, where avoidance of short-term emotional distress in persons served is a by-product of unilateral "expert" decisions, often superficially justified by the best interest standard.

Brief Scenario: Dr. Melanie Black, a rehabilitation psychologist, works in an outpatient rehabilitation clinic, performing evaluations and providing treatment for patients who have continuing needs after completing inpatient rehabilitation. Her colleague, Dr. Antoinette "Toni" Fouisse, is a part-time consultant to the rehabilitation program, conducting vocational evaluations and supporting the work readiness program. Melanie has noticed that Toni, on several occasions, has made excuses to avoid providing services to patients without insurance funding for those services. The expectation of the organization for which the psychologists worked is that persons in financial need are provided services, with flexible financial plans arranged via the business office. However, a financial incentive program is also operating that rewards professional staff with bonuses when their collections exceed benchmark levels in any given quarter. Toni has been a regular recipient of bonuses over the past year.

Brief Commentary: The rehabilitation psychologist's **ethical obligation** is to attempt to informally address what appears to be an ethical problem with her colleague. The assumption is that the observing psychologist has ample reason to believe that there has been an **ethical breach**. In this example, Dr. Fouisse has presented no hard evidence of professional practice problems. Instead, she appears to be "cherry picking" funded patients, passing over those individuals without funding, thereby shunting them to her colleagues. This business strategy is reflected in varying degrees throughout the for-profit health care system, where patients with health insurance are served according to health need, while economically disadvantaged individuals with equivalent health needs, but no funding, are referred to indigent care organizations or Medicaid provider organizations (if they qualify)—with no guarantee of or incentive for adequate service provision.

It is important to note that the organization for which Drs. Black and Fouisse work has a policy regarding persons with financial need being flexibly served by the business office. However, this policy is rather vaguely described, and could potentially rule out service provision for an indigent person. The troublesome aspect of this case, from the ethical perspective, is that a psychologist appears to be informally screening out economically disadvantaged patients on the basis of financial criteria for personal financial gain, independent of the organization's policy. An unrecognized **conflict of interest** occurs because Toni's objectivity may be affected by her personal financial interest and the potential monetary advantage she gains by denying that service.

Dr. Black's ethical obligation is to attempt to clarify her perception of her colleague's behavior—seeking an **informal resolution** of a potential ethical violation. Presenting a rationale for economically screening patients may prove to be a topic that spurs meaningful conversation. However, defensive denial of wrongdoing simply increases suspicion of an ethical problem. The fulcrum around which the perceived ethical breach turns is Dr. Fouisse's receipt of financial reward for her high proportion of successful collections, as compared with her colleagues. Comparing work productivity across psychology staff (e.g., gathering data on hours worked, numbers of patients seen, types of charges generated) can help in clarifying this type of difficult discussion. **Accuracy** in discussion of this issue is paramount, as are the implications of a **violation of trust** among the psychology staff at this imbalance in treatment assignment.

Dr. Black would also be ethically bound to explore the organization's incentive program policy, by providing administrators the example cited above. Incentive policies are typically designed to **equitably** encourage increased staff productivity, thereby benefiting both the staff person and the organization. It would be counterproductive (not to mention legally risky) for a health care organization to economically discriminate against health service consumers, even if unintentionally. Consequences of such examples as that described above often result in amendments to incentive policies.

RELEVANT STANDARDS

2.03 Conflicts between Ethics and Organizational Demands
2.04 Informal Resolution of Ethical Violations
3.06 Conflict of Interest
6.04 Fees and Financial Arrangements

5   Principle: Justice

JUSTICE IS DEFINED as fair and equitable access to and benefit from (rehabilitation) psychology services and research by all persons, ensuring quality in all processes and procedures offered (APA, 2002). In the bioethics literature (e.g., Beauchamp & Childress, 2009), the principle of justice is most often employed in guiding health care policy decisions regarding developing accessible systems of health care delivery and ensuring equity when allocating scarce resources. Instead of emphasizing overall good or harm, justice focuses on the fair allocation and distribution of resources. In other words, justice influences the distribution of potential benefits and harm. Examples of relevant questions in this context might include: How much treatment time do I schedule with each patient? In what manner are specific treatment services apportioned within a treatment session? Does the patient's level of engagement influence allocation of my services? Can I ethically avoid patients who cannot pay for services?

Emphasis is often placed on meeting the needs of special populations (e.g., persons with disabilities, underserved populations, etc.). However, defining these needs can be complicated, and this position assumes that need is the critical variable on which resource distribution is decided. Does need receive greatest priority weighting? Do those who seem to deserve the resources actually receive greatest priority? On the surface this latter question might not seem a reasonable consideration from a rehabilitation perspective, but what if one defines "deserving" as patient effort. We can and do allocate our services in the interest of those who can use them the most based on their engagement in the rehabilitation process. That said, if one rehabilitation patient is expending less effort in treatment than another, is it a just decision to spend less treatment time with that person? Perhaps they actually need more treatment time, but apportioned to address barriers to effort expenditure.

Most psychologists would agree that we have a fiduciary responsibility to our patients (i.e., providing appropriate care). However, as mentioned previously, in the United States health care is not considered an absolute right, and the patient is not necessarily the only one with a vested interest in just care. Witness the family, the organization, and several potential others (e.g., other team members, employers, claims agents, etc.) who create social, policy, and regulatory pressure regarding allocation decisions. Offering pro bono services falls under the purview of the Ethics Code standards, but this moral obligation must be balanced against the immediate costs to the provider and risk to the viability of professional service provision into the future.

From an ethical perspective, conflicts of interest also fall broadly within the concept of justice. Conflicts of interest are not inherently unethical. It is one's response to the conflicts that determines the ethical soundness in a given situation. But how do we reconcile our duty to one patient versus another patient, or our responsibilities to others with vested interests? We may not consciously think about it all the time, but psychologists make these types of decisions every day. In answering these questions, one must understand the ethical, legal, social, and organizational dynamics that interact with patient progression, the varied needs of the patient, family, and community. A key responsibility is to make decisions such that one's basis for those decisions would be viewed as reasonable by one's peers, given similar circumstances (i.e., the reasonable person standard employed in ethics and legal judgments). In this chapter, we will drill down to the level of the individual rehabilitation psychologist, exploring justice as it influences everyday clinical service delivery and the research enterprise.

CASE EXAMPLE 5.1

"But, I can't afford it...."

I. Quick Reference
Critical Incident

Tina Woods, an actress with a small theatrical road company, had been injured in a motor vehicle crash, sustaining significant orthopedic and deforming facial injuries. Her automobile insurance medical coverage was authorized for subacute rehabilitation treatment. Dr. Bill Cash, the rehabilitation psychologist consulting to the subacute program, had provided an initial evaluation and had begun treatment.

However, shortly after the patient transitioned to the subacute rehabilitation environment, the medical benefits available, including those for psychological services, had been quickly exhausted. A legal case was pending, with a contingency provision for delayed service fee reimbursement. The consulting psychologist was faced with a decision whether to continue services with an individual without financial resources to pay for that care.

Emotional adjustment needs of the patient were acute, given her livelihood depended to a great extent on her appearance and physical abilities. Both aspects of her personal and professional identity had been abruptly and tragically altered as a result of her injuries. The patient had been eager to work with the rehabilitation psychologist after the initial evaluation findings and treatment plan were explained. However, the psychologist had been having significant difficulty making his consulting business a viable enterprise in the context of a weak economy and poor mental health insurance reimbursement rates. Consequently, he was reluctant to take on another pro bono case. While the health care facility had policy provisions for indigent care, this safety net did not extend to the psychologist's contractual arrangement with the organization. Thus, the rehabilitation psychologist opted to refer the patient for alternative mental health services offered within the organization. The premature service termination resulted in a significant negative emotional reaction from the patient that made the likelihood of her utilizing alternative service providers very low.

If the rehabilitation psychologist had consulted you regarding what to do, would you have agreed with his decision? As you weigh the issues, take into consideration the following questions.

- What services, if any, do you think the rehabilitation psychologist is obligated to provide this patient under his contract with the subacute rehabilitation center?
- Are there circumstances under which a psychologist can refuse to provide nonreimbursed care?
- What steps should psychologists take to proactively address financial disadvantage issues with patients?
- What are the organizational policies and obligations regarding provision of indigent care?
- What steps should be taken to appropriately terminate care?

TABLE 5.1
CASE ANALYSIS SUMMARY

Ethical Principles	Relevant Standards	Context & Key Stakeholders	Organizational & Legal Issues	Alternative Solutions
I. Primary Justice - All patients admitted to rehabilitation facilities have the right to access needed psychological services; the RP is obligated to resolve the funding problem with NRI administration in order to avoid inequitable care delivery based solely on ability to pay II. Secondary Beneficence and Nonmaleficence - Denial of needed services could increase the likelihood of emotional harm to the patient; provision of services would likely enhance adjustment to disability - If psychologist continues services without reimbursement, he may have to cancel the contract resulting in at least short-term harm to patients Responsibility - inadequate negotiation of consulting contract to address indigent care - lack of responsibility to address financial needs of patient	3.01 Unfair discrimination - Failure to provide needed service due to financial limits could be considered socioeconomic discrimination 3.04 Avoiding Harm - the psychologist must appropriately manage termination 3.06 Conflict of Interest - If payment is linked to lawsuit outcome, bias could be introduced into treatment 3.10 Informed consent - Information should be provided about financial responsibilities at the start of treatment 3.12 Interruption of services - RP must make provisions for service delivery if treatment is interrupted secondary to financial limitations 10.10 Terminating Therapy - Premature termination for financial reasons requires arrangements be made to meet patient needs	- Patient—presents with psychological and physical needs that require treatment - RP—obligated to provide services per NRI contract - Patient's mother—supports her daughter's need for funding via litigation, NRI Administration -Policy for charity care does not currently cover consultant reimbursement; collegial cooperation regarding funded referrals a consideration Private legal team - Outcome of lawsuit may allow delayed funding for psychological services; but only if the suit obtains a ruling in favor of the complainant	- Organizational policy and procedure at NRI—indigent care and state allocation of funds does not account for financial nonpayment of consultant fees, indirectly jeopardizing continuing services - A negligence-based lawsuit was filed in Common Pleas court with the city identified as the defendant and the patient as the plaintiff; seeking medical expenses and damages; not likely to be settled for years	A. Provide pro bono services after funding exhausted per patient need B. Provide pro bono services through rehab admission; then, arrange outpatient follow-up options C. Terminate treatment after auto insurance funds exhausted D. Arrange for counseling support services through other hospital resources E. Continue providing service; renegotiate NRI contract or seek policy change to deal with indigent care for MH needs

Resolutions

A. **Provide pro bono services after funding is exhausted**

   Pro

   a) *Service delivery continued per patient need; meets patient expectations; includes RP responsibility for arranging outpatient follow-up services, as needed*
   b) *Pro bono service provision per Ethics Code, justified by patient need*
   c) *Psychologist fulfills responsibility to patient, based on initial evaluation results, to provide treatment after having failed to consider financial issues at the outset—concept of due care*
   d) *Treatment mission of HCO upheld regarding service provision to all patients admitted*

   Con

   a) *Financial burden placed on RP for services delivered*
   b) *Pattern of increasing financial loss secondary to declining insurance reimbursement; indicator of dysfunctional consultation contract*
   c) *Patient responsibility for payment of health care fees is circumvented*

B. **Provide pro bono services throughout rehabilitation admission; then, arrange outpatient follow-up—Preferred (also see E)**

   Pro

   a) *Service delivery per expectations within consultancy contract for inpatient rehabilitation patient*
   b) *Proper hand-off to community-based follow-up outpatient services per contract*
   c) *Provides some time for psychologist to address patient's anxiety regarding transfer of care*
   d) *The patient must confront personal responsibility for needed outpatient services*

   Con

   a) *Financial burden on the psychologist for this case; reflects a continuing negative reimbursement trend that threatens contract viability*
   b) *Further (financial, emotional) stress on patient at a time of outpatient transition; confronting the reality of limited national health system "safety net" provisions for indigent care*
   c) *Ignores need for longer-term resolution for future referrals*

C. **Terminate treatment after funding exhausted**

   Pro

   a) *Relieves financial burden for this case; passively counters negative reimbursement trend*

Con
a) *Ignores patient's inpatient and outpatient needs, and inconsistent with patient's expectations based in initial subacute evaluation data and subsequent treatment plan generation*
b) *Ignores valid exercise of pro bono solution via Ethics Code standards*
c) *Violates spirit of consultancy contract for service provision for all patients referred*

D. **Arrange counseling services through other hospital resources**
Pro
a) *Attempts to meet patient needs via utilization of alternate HCO resources*
b) *Passively relieves immediate financial burden on RP for unreimbursed care*
c) *Attempts to balance realistic financial pressures with transfer of care options*

Con
a) *Involves transfer of service delivery for purely financial, rather than quality of care reasons*
b) *Violates patient treatment expectations established during initial evaluation*
c) *Ignores pro bono solution, having begun the treatment relationship*
d) *No guarantee that alternative HCPs possess comparable skills or that services will be available simultaneous with care termination*

E. **Provide care and seek rehabilitation facility policy change, agree with legal contingency for funding—Preferred (also see B)**
Pro
a) *Provision of needed services with delayed contingency plan; allows for pro bono service delivery if the legal settlement is not forthcoming*
b) *Attempts to meet long-term financial needs of RP for this case, even if delayed*
c) *Provides for potential HCO contractual negotiations toward a more equitable financial arrangement regarding indigent care; parallel to other rehabilitation disciplines (employees)*
d) *Given the legal alternative payment method, the patient is indirectly responsible for payment of health care charges*

Con
a) *No provision of short-term reimbursement for RP to keep the contract viable*
b) *Contractual/policy negotiations with HCO will delay a short-term solution to the RP's financial dilemma*

II. Contextual Influences

Twenty-six year-old Tina Woods, the lead in a small professional theater road company production, was on her way to a cast party when her car hit a patch of black ice and spun out of control. Ms. Woods's vehicle struck a tree, resulting in multitrauma orthopedic injuries and significant facial lacerations. Fortunately, Tina was spared a traumatic brain injury by virtue of a flawlessly functioning restraint system. However, her uninterrupted conscious state during the prolonged extraction from her mangled vehicle took an emotional toll. Tina spent 2 weeks in Suburban Medical Center, undergoing surgical fixation of both upper arms and her left leg, as well as the first of several planned plastic surgeries to cosmetically repair her facial lacerations. Because she was rendered non-weight-bearing in three extremities, Tina was transferred to Northeastern Rehabilitation Institute (NRI) for limited subacute rehabilitation and caregiving training for her mother, Sue Woods. With no health insurance benefits offered by the theater company, her automobile insurance policy's personal injury medical coverage was Tina's sole source of medical payment, but was nearly exhausted from her acute hospital stay.

Three days into her NRI admission, members of Tina's rehabilitation treatment team had observed Tina quietly crying at times in her treatment sessions. This emotional reaction was most acute whenever a mirror was used to visually reinforce proper trunk balance and transfer techniques. Tina's mood did not brighten when the members of the team had tried in vain to cheer her up with supportive comments during social conversation. A physical therapist had seen one of Tina's recent play performances and provided effusive praise regarding Tina's ability to light up an entire stage. Unfortunately, this comment lit up Tina in quite the wrong direction. Consequently, news of Tina's emotional distress made its way to the program's consulting rehabilitation psychologist, Dr. William "Bill" Cash. Dr. Cash was in private practice in the local community and provided services to several subacute rehabilitation programs, including the program at NRI. His consulting contract with NRI specified that he bill for clinical services provided through his private practice. Additionally, Dr. Cash was paid a small administrative stipend to participate in meetings and provide continuing professional education in-services to the NRI staff.

Upon receiving the referral, Dr. Cash reviewed the electronic health record and then arranged a meeting with Tina. During the initial evaluation, she was dysphoric about her painful injuries and the loss of functional independence. Tina's additional emotional burden was the "horrific transformation" of her facial appearance. Her pessimistic self-assessment saw her hope for a continuing career as an actress beginning to dissipate. Based on initial evaluation findings, the psychologist's treatment plan consisted of individual therapy sessions three times per week, and a once per week disability adjustment group session, cofacilitated by Bill and the unit's social worker. Both interventions were projected through Tina's 14-day stay at NRI. Tina's initial engagement with the treatment process was positive, and she showed promise for achieving emotional stability prior to discharge. However, at the end of her first week at NRI, Dr. Cash and the rehab team were informed that Tina's auto insurance–based medical coverage had run out. With this harsh reality in mind, Dr. Cash reluctantly informed Tina that, as a result of her insurance limitations, he would no longer be able to provide her with psychological services… that is, unless she could pay out-of-pocket, or had another source of financial support. Tina was predictably devastated by the news, and expressed pointed anger that a psychologist would "abandon" a patient already in treatment for financial reasons.

Later that day, Dr. Cash was phoned by Sue Woods, Tina's mother, who said that she too was disappointed in the treatment discontinuance. However, she had a possible resolution to the problem. She intended to bring litigation against the city for negligence regarding inadequate signage on a winding road, well known for being hazardous in adverse weather, and failure to adequately salt that section of road. She asked if Dr. Cash would continue to work with Tina, with future payment linked to a lien on any proceeds from the lawsuit. Bill Cash said that he would seriously consider the offer, and would make a decision the following day.

There was a broader negative factor influencing this situation. Dr. Cash had experienced a 24% drop in consulting revenues across the varied rehabilitation programs he served during the 6 months prior to Tina Woods's admission to NRI. This had occurred despite a steady stream of appropriate referrals. In response to increasing insurance "carve-outs" for mental health services to individuals with medical diagnoses, Dr. Cash had transformed his community private practice into an out-of-pocket enterprise. To say that he was struggling was putting it mildly. Northeastern Rehabilitation Institute, pursuant to its commitment to the underserved community, was admitting indigent patients with increasing regularity. The state provided annual funds to HCOs in order to partially offset costs of such policies, helping to soften the financial burden. Notably, these funds were not available to private consultants. In a conversation with the attending physician at NRI, Dr. Cash requested referrals of insured patients. While agreeing to this strategy in principle, both men acknowledged the moral duty of HCPs within NRI to "treat all comers," reflecting the organization's policy. These financial realities weighed on Bill Cash as he considered Tina Woods's situation.

The following partial solutions to the financial challenge were considered by the rehabilitation psychologist. He could provide as-needed services under the proposed contingent lien against a legal settlement (i.e., payment substantially delayed and not guaranteed). Alternatively, he could provide services pro bono, adding further to his financial woes. Additionally, he could request one-time financial support from NRI administration—risking administrative rejection, or conversely opening a door for future contract negotiations containing a potential remedy in such cases. Finally, he could transfer services to the organization's social services and/or chaplaincy personnel. However, some of these individuals were not expressly trained in evaluating and treating the special needs of persons with disabilities. No matter which of the potential resolutions selected, Dr. Cash would provide an appropriate community referral to continue treatment past the point of discharge from NRI. Upon presenting the possible resolutions to the financial limitations problem to Tina Woods for her preferences, the rehabilitation psychologist was summarily rebuffed by the patient, who refused to have anything to do with him or his plans. Tina adamantly refused any further contact with Dr. Cash at NRI or afterward, and asked him to leave her presence immediately.

Feeling terrible about the patient's rejection of his good faith offers, Dr. Cash actively pursued the list of qualified mental health resources in the community, and presented this list to both the patient and Sue Woods prior to Tina's discharge from NRI. He hoped that Tina would reconsider seeking treatment after residing for a time in the community. However, the silent steely glare that Tina focused on Dr. Cash as she was wheeled from the facility did not reinforce that hope.

Commentary

Dr. Cash was faced with multiple challenges in this case, the majority of which involved his own missteps, placing his compliance with Ethics Code standards associated with the principles of justice and responsibility in jeopardy. The practical realities of declining service reimbursement are clearly raising the financial burden on HCOs, psychologists, and patients alike. However, this burden does not exonerate the psychologist from his or her ethical obligations regarding managing patient care decisions, including payment for services planned or rendered. Having failed (1) to explore Tina's funding resources upon receiving the referral, (2) to adequately inform Tina about his consultant status related to how finances were managed, and (3) to negotiate financial arrangements for his services prior to beginning evaluation and treatment, Dr. Cash was left with limited options in attempting to regain ethical footing, none of which was ideal. The end result of his omissions was harm to the patient and, at least in the short-term, to the discipline of psychology given the patient's tainted view of the profession resulting in her refusal to seek continuing services. In addition, if Dr. Cash knowingly limited or terminated service primarily for financial reasons, especially after initiating treatment without fulfilling his ethical obligations to address the patient's financial circumstances, the patient could legitimately consider his actions as unfair discrimination based on her socioeconomic status (conflicting with Ethics Standard 3.01). Although the Ethics Code allows for interruption of services secondary to financial limitations (Ethics Standard 3.12), in this case it appears that the financial circumstances could have been clarified earlier, which would have allowed the psychologist to weigh financial information in adaptive treatment planning discussions with the patient. In addition, he may have had specific contractual obligations to provide nonreimbursed care as part of his services to NRI. This point would need further clarification. Finally, there was no evidence that Tina, despite her emotionality, was incompetent to participate in a discussion regarding fees. Given the psychologist independently billed for services, and unless otherwise specified in the contract, it was Dr. Cash's professional obligation to reach an agreement with the patient regarding compensation (see Ethics Standard 6.04). If this discussion had occurred, perhaps the patient's mother would have become financially engaged earlier in the process.

Based on the events of this case, an adaptive approach to resolution is a combination of alternatives B and E from Table 5.1. When patients present with legitimate rehabilitation psychology service needs, the issue of payment for services needs to be addressed as a secondary priority behind provision of services. This prioritization is especially noted in the context of contract services provided in rehabilitation programs, where the integrated team treatment approach should not be compromised by financial constraints. Admission to such facilities comes under the tacit assumption on the part of the patient/family that all warranted services will be provided. If a rehabilitation psychologist consultant provides services within the team context, and billing occurs through that person's private practice, a predictable and transparent mechanism for communicating such an arrangement should exist, and be integrated into the consent to treat discussion and signed by the patient/surrogate at admission.

In addressing the broader policy implications in this case, Dr. Cash's planned contract renegotiations should address the steadily increasing trend of indigent/charity care admissions at NRI. An equitable plan to distribute financial resources, and to provide adequate care for those individuals incapable of paying for needed services, should be established within the consultancy contract. Such an approach may include a stable monthly contract payment for services rendered within a specified number of hours per week/month, the result of bundling psychological service charges with rehabilitation team treatment charges. Alternatively, the organization could opt to employ the rehabilitation psychologist, who could then indirectly share in the state appropriations funds disbursed to HCOs for indigent care cost offsets, with charges similarly bundled. It may also be advantageous for an employed rehabilitation psychologist's service charges to be unbundled and billed independently by the rehabilitation facility to cover salary and benefits. The viability of any of the above alternatives will vary by state and organization.

Finally, the psychologist did make a constructive decision to mitigate the harm by providing options for alternative sources of care, rather than simply dropping the case altogether. In general, if termination of services becomes warranted for financial reasons, the psychologist may still meet his or her ethical obligations by providing alternative care options after discussion with the patient regarding the transitional process. Given the patient's refusal of treatment, Dr. Cash's effort and encouragement to connect his patient with community-based counseling services partially addresses the problem of questionable service termination. Employing that approach places the decision to engage with follow-up services with the patient. However, as noted previously, the negative experience that Tina Woods had with the rehabilitation psychologist would likely skew her decision-making. Assuming that the patient will reside with Sue Woods after discharge, additional opportunities to seek out therapeutic services in the community may arise, reinforcing the importance of referral information being provided.

Disposition

Tina Woods was discharged from NRI to her mother's home. Sue Woods, concerned for her daughter's physical and emotional health, withdrew monies from her own retirement fund to pay for outpatient rehabilitation therapies. However, Tina steadfastly refused to become involved with psychological treatment, citing her disillusionment with the profession while an inpatient. Sue Woods bided her time regarding her conviction that Tina would, at some undefined point in time, require more psychological treatment. In the meantime, Tina and her mother, as cosignatory, took out a loan to pay for Tina's proposed plastic surgeries under a payment plan negotiated with an outpatient surgical center. Tina was convinced that such treatment would be her ticket to resuming her stage career, the only occupation she had known since graduating from college.

After several months and four reconstructive facial surgeries, Tina felt that she was ready to return to her touring theater company. She was emotionally buoyed by her surgeon's encouragement after admiring his handiwork during her last follow-up visit. By that time the play in which Tina had starred had completed its run, and the artistic director had been replaced. Tina immediately auditioned for the female lead in an upcoming light comedy-musical production, a part that she considered herself well-suited to win. However, she failed to secure any part following the audition. Tina received disheartening feedback from the casting director, indicating that her altered appearance would not be amenable to "audience sensitivities." The casting director, who was also new to the company, rather harshly suggested that Tina try to tackle darker, macabre roles, in which her physical attributes could be displayed to Tina's advantage. This event marked the first time that Tina had failed to secure a spot in a production that she had seriously pursued. This blow to her emotional reserves, delivered by her professional peers, was significant.

Crushed by the experience, Tina returned to her mother's home, feeling both dejected and a failure. It was Sue Woods, ever sympathetic to the struggles of her children, who finally convinced her daughter to seek long-overdue psychological services, and this time Tina relented. The list of rehabilitation-savvy community providers Dr. Cash had given Tina and her mother months earlier was finally put to its intended use. The fact that Tina did not pursue her treatment abandonment claim with the State Board of Psychology was a fortunate happenstance for Dr. Bill Cash.

Learning Opportunities

1. What proactive measures do you incorporate into your professional activities to ensure that equity is an integral part of your practice?
2. How can you evaluate the adequacy/fairness of operational strategies of the health care, educational, and/or research organizations with whom you are allied?

Brief Scenario: Dr. Robin Melandri is a grant-funded rehabilitation researcher specializing in addressing rehabilitation psychology research questions. Robin is under contract with a health research organization that recently partnered with a pharmaceutical company (providing a much-needed infusion of capital) to investigate a new treatment for reducing the cytotoxic cascade associated with new-onset central nervous system injury. Dr. Melandri's arm of the study is to evaluate the potential quality of life impact of the proposed treatment in persons with acute brain and/or spinal cord injuries. The treatment regimen is extremely complex—in terms of the administration time window and time-consuming repeated treatment with long infusion durations. In addition, the side effects observed to date have been serious in some cases—but not serious enough for the researchers or Internal Review Board (IRB) to consider terminating the project. During the informed consent process (with patients and proxies when capacity was impaired), Dr. Melandri discovered that many of the recruited individuals who otherwise met study criteria could not readily grasp the complexities, intent, and potential benefits and risks of the study as explained during the scripted verbal and written informed consent. When she expressed this concern to the Principle Investigator (PI) and administrators of the research organization, they told her to stop recruiting "those people" (indicating individuals who struggled with comprehending the underlying concepts under investigation) and to focus on people who could readily understand the collective vision of the study. The upshot of this comment, on further inquiry, was that the hoped-for beneficiaries of the study would be those people who would demonstrate stronger pharmacological effect, incur less CNS insult, and have a greater chance of contributing in substantial ways to society in the future.

Brief Commentary: Dr. Melandri is faced with a complex challenge. As a rehabilitation psychologist researcher, she is bound by the Ethics Code to pursue **informal resolution** of apparent **unfair discrimination** by another psychologist. While we are unaware of the professions of the project PI and research organization administrator, bioethical breaches such as the discriminatory bias in biomedical research protocols described above warrant an effort toward resolution. Otherwise, the psychologist's action (or inaction) passively reinforces a discriminatory process. Indeed, the assumption that an individual who struggles with comprehension of complex research methodology would be less likely to contribute meaningfully to society than a person able to understand the existing informed consent information is without merit.

Dr. Melandri faces potential political risks in pursuing this obligatory informal resolution. It is hoped that both the PI and administrator would respond in an open manner to a well-crafted argument to broaden the participant pool to individuals who require accommodations during the consenting process. Indeed, a competency desired in all rehabilitation psychologists is **advocating for individuals with disabilities**. Therefore, modifying the consent procedure to enhance understanding of the research project rationale, along with benefits and risks of participation, would be the proper resolution.

If the key players react to her ethically cautionary message in a defensive manner, expressing unwillingness to alter the problematic participant consent material or process, Dr. Melandri should consider recusing herself from the project. However, such a decision could put her position within the organization in jeopardy, and the biased study would move forward with another willing investigator. Although the Ethics Code provides some protection for an individual coming forward with an ethical concern, this protection exists within the psychologists' code and may not apply across disciplines. The **refusal of a key stakeholder** in an ethical conflict to participate in rectifying the problem cannot serve as a deterrent to problem resolution. In such a situation, Dr. Melandri may consider pleading her case to the organization's IRB. Since this nationally required review mechanism within all research enterprises is structured under federal regulations, biased or discriminatory participant selection should not be tolerated, even if discovered after a study has been initiated. This research project is funded, at least in part by a private entity (pharmaceutical company), so NIH research ethics standards may not be directly enforceable. Nonetheless, the tenets of NIH standards would certainly lend credibility to Dr. Melandri's arguments against discriminatory participant selection. Another source of potential leverage would be seeking guidance from pertinent state health profession licensing boards, all of whom have ethics committees appended. In any case, tolerance of discriminatory practices in conducting human research cannot be justified.

The reader's awareness and consideration of a broad range of **potential consequences of** seeking **informal resolution** of ethical conflicts cannot be overemphasized. This awareness should drive information gathering and peer consultation during the planning process before any action is taken toward adaptive and constructive resolution.

RELEVANT STANDARDS

1.04 Informal Resolution of Ethical Violations
1.08 Unfair Discrimination against Complainants and Respondents
3.01 Unfair Discrimination
3.04 Avoiding Harm
8.02 (b) Informed Consent to Research
8.08 (a) Debriefing

CASE EXAMPLE 5.2

"But it's the only available health care...."

I. Quick Reference

Critical Incident

Dr. Jenny Yankovic, a rehabilitation psychologist with international field research experience has been hired as a consultant to a research team initiating a project focusing on the treatment of neuropathic pain in individuals with limb amputations. Despite the team having received IRB approval, the psychologist has serious concerns about the possibility of inappropriate incentives or inducements being offered to the participants by the study's sponsor, a medical equipment development firm. The coprincipal investigators, Drs. Vetch and Dietrich, believe the project should move forward without delay because all required approvals to conduct the study have been acquired.

The rehabilitation psychologist's concerns highlight the possibility of social and/or physical harm coming to those who choose to participate in the project, which is proposed to be implemented in several third-world refugee camps (an efficient use of a relevant convenience sample). Additionally, the psychologist is concerned that there may be subtle coercion applied if the population under study is subject to poor health care service provision in the social context of the refugee camps. In some cases, individuals desiring participation may see the research project as their only means of access to health care services, and those not meeting inclusion criteria may be denied this access. This perception is made even more likely because there is a physical examination included in the protocol.

As a rehabilitation psychologist and consulting scientist on this project, consider the types of information you would like to know before being comfortable proceeding on the project. As part of your deliberations, consider the following questions.

- What types of undue influence might occur regarding consent when research protocols include the provision of services desired by the potential study participants?
- What steps can be taken to minimize coercion when soliciting consent from vulnerable populations who need or can greatly benefit from health services offered as part of the research protocol?
- What protections can the psychologist recommend to avoid unintended secondary outcomes?
- Under what circumstances, if any, is it appropriate to initiate human trials on specific vulnerable populations when broader participation is feasible?
- What steps can be taken to protect participant confidentiality in research in which participants may be easily identified by the tightly integrated communities in which they live?
- What types of additional considerations, if any, are necessary when assessing level of participant risk in vulnerable populations?

Resolutions

    A. ***Implement study as originally planned***

                                      Pro

        a) *Causes least delay in beginning the project*
        b) *Stays within budget*
        c) *Provides beneficial health evaluation more quickly than delayed study initiation*

TABLE 5.2
CASE ANALYSIS SUMMARY

Ethical Principles	Relevant Standards	Context & Key Stakeholders	Organizational & Legal Issues	Alternative Solutions
I. Primary Justice - Ethical concepts of undue profit and inducement apply II. Secondary Beneficence & Nonmaleficence - While benefit potential exists for the treatment, so does risk of social backlash because of incentive strategy used Fidelity & Responsibility - The RP researcher must proactively advocate for participant protections in accord with ethical research tenets	8.06(a) Offering inducements for research participation - avoid excessive or inappropriate financial or other inducements when there is risk of coercion 8.06(b) - When services are involved, care must be taken to clarify nature, risks, obligations, and limitations of such services 8.04(a) - RP must take steps to protect the prospective participants from adverse consequences for declining or withdrawing from participation 8.02(a.4.) - Need to inform participants of reasonably foreseeable factors that may influence willingness to participate	RP—advocates for ethical protections Research co-PI—pushes medical incentives Research co-PI —wants to address aims of study and ethical issues Company Representative— has interests of his company as primary motivation Epidemiology Consultant— Agrees with participant protections Research Field Coordinators— have personal experience supporting participant protections for participants; previous work with RP	- Published research ethics guidelines and required agency certifications emphasize participant protections - IRB in place to ensure participant protections and ethical research; variability in review processes across institutions and agencies - International law and national laws govern external research activities; variable requirements and enforcement	A. Stick with original time frame and IRB-approved protections B. Delay study in order to survey social factors influencing participants C. Simultaneously survey participant population regarding ethical protections while the study is in progress D. Send an advance team to survey the population regarding participant protections; alert IRB to changes in incentive plan and participant protections

Con

a) *Ignores ethical concerns regarding patient protections*
b) *Provides tacit approval for corporate constituency on the team to exert unbalanced influence over the project's logistical operations*

  c) *Violates NIH research ethics standards regarding identified needs for patient protections*
  d) *Potentially compromises scientific goals of the study by introducing risk of social bias*
 B. ***Delay study in order to survey social factors influencing participants***
        Pro
  a) *Allows for evaluation of potential modifications to the study to enhance patient protections*
  b) *Supports social contextual basis for any patient protection modifications to come from survey data*
        Con
  a) *Delays project beyond optimal time frame per original research proposal*
  b) *Does not account for further IRB delays regarding any potential method modifications*
  c) *Does not specify patient protections required to address ethical concerns*
 C. ***Survey participant population regarding ethical protections while originally designed study in progress***
        Pro
  a) *Allows study to proceed along original time line; saves time if no bias identified*
  b) *Supports team dialogue regarding ethical issues*
  c) *Addresses, in part, ethical concerns regarding patient protections and potential social bias in results*
        Con
  a) *Risks invalidating data collection if survey results reveal social bias in participants*
  b) *Post hoc manipulation of data to correct for social bias weakens scientific integrity of original design*
  c) *Altering method would require additional IRB review—delaying time line*
  d) *Unidentified risk of participant harm if needed ethical protections not in place at study initiation*
 D. ***Send advance team to survey population regarding participant protections, inform IRB of incentive plan and participant protection changes—Preferred***
        Pro
  a) *Allows ethical concerns to be addressed prior to beginning study*
  b) *Allows for IRB review of any required modifications to method via survey data*

c) *Allows for scientific integrity of the project by supporting patient protections*

Con

a) *Funding costs increased for medical equipment company sponsor*
b) *Project delayed from original time line; study agreement could potentially unravel*
c) *Delays potential medical benefit*

II. Contextual Influences

The cast of players in the meeting to discuss this research project was impressive. The consultants included Dr. Jenny Yankovic (rehabilitation psychologist), Dr. Matt Ortlieb (MegaMed engineer and company representative—manufacturer of the equipment under investigation), and Dr. Seth Yamato (epidemiologist). Drs. Wili Vetch (physiatrist) and Johnny Dietrich (biomedical engineer) were project co-PIs, while Lisa Voit and Bobby Melton functioned as field research coordinators. With the exception of the experimental equipment developer's representative, Matt Ortlieb, Jenny had worked in the past with each of the professionals on the project. She respected both their credentials and demonstrated expertise.

The project in question was designed to gather the first human trial data on a new electromagnetic stimulation (EM) device intended to treat neuropathic pain associated with new limb amputations. Matt presented a product update, emphasizing the design changes related to EM signal frequency and duration and the shape of the emitter head that were expected to produce more consistently reproducible data than the earlier model. The field coordinators then described the results of a recruiting trip to one of the refugee camps in Africa. Under the protection of a UN Peacekeeper force in the region, Bobby and Lisa had been able to visit several camps where potential research participants (individuals with limb amputations from regional civil wars) were initially screened. The estimates looked optimistic regarding obtaining the number of participants to meet statistical power requirements.

Jenny began to feel that she would become the unwelcome social conscience of the group when she laid the details of her serious ethical concerns regarding undue inducement and undue profit linked to the project. The research project description that she had reviewed proposed a participation incentive involving payment of a modest amount of money to each participant, with that scenario repeated across the 10 proposed treatment trials. Despite the multitrial accrual of funds by participants who endured to project completion, the total amounted to a relatively small sum, even when tied to the living standards of the recruits. This sum was then compared with the projected profits that MegaMed stood to make from the sale of the project. Jenny added another concern about potentially biasing project results by only selecting participants who were economically and socially disadvantaged. She readily acknowledged that the strategy of utilizing residents of refugee camps, where the incidence of individuals with amputations was amply in excess of the general population, was a strategically efficient bonus. Nonetheless, the caution regarding population bias potentially skewing results and restricting generalization of the data still applied, and needed to be addressed in the experimental design.

Jenny then presented her final concern—the inclusion of a full medical exam and basic preventative treatment in the project's participation incentive package. She explained that the screening data presented by the field coordinators suggested that most of the potential recruits did not have adequate access to proper medical care. Being involved in the study would give the participants, simply by virtue of their tragic injuries, an unintended social advantage over the other residents in the refugee camps—perhaps putting those people at risk of social ostracism, or worse… personal danger.

Needless to say, the committee erupted into verbal chaos when Jenny had completed her presentation. She had diligently tried to gear her remarks toward encouraging study modification, rather than pushing the train off the tracks. When asked for clarification, Jenny gave an example. When the study cited the payment per treatment session as a monetary amount, there was no explanation of how that amount was determined. Paying too little for participation makes the study attractive to only the lowest social classes. Paying too high an amount would likely result in exclusion of the most economically disadvantaged classes, in favor of middle and even upper classes—although the chances of individuals from that social rung being in refugee camps was admittedly low. So, arriving at the contextually accurate amount must result from a survey of monetary resources available to the camps' participant groups, producing a data-driven decision that could stand scrutiny. Jenny's epidemiology consultant colleague Seth added support for her concerns, asking the investigators for an analysis of the effects of access to health evaluation and preventative treatment on those related to the potential participants, and those individuals residing in proximity to the participants. The latter group may become aware of the health care boon provided the participants, but would lack an adequate reason for a possible misperception of favoritism.

The ensuing discussion then focused on undesirable delays in beginning this human trial, especially after having had numerous IRB meetings to deal with other methodological criticisms. The group tried in vain to recall just how the details of the decision to incentivize the participants had been reached, eventually concluding that sufficient, contextually valid due diligence had not been performed. The discussion then turned to offering health evaluation and basic preventative treatment to participants. Dr. Vetch shared her personal experience in Doctors Without Borders, where access to health evaluation and basic treatment was viewed as unequivocally beneficial of underserved peoples. She added that very few individuals residing in regional civil war refugee camps overseen by UN peacekeepers had adequate medical care on a consistent basis. Too many were transient. Too many refused care equitably provided to members of social groups with whom they were in conflict, and too many did not trust Western health care providers. She ended by emphasizing the need to retain that incentive in the research protocol to screen for potential confounding medical conditions that could result in the team dumping otherwise solid data.

Lisa, one of the field coordinators, added that she had witnessed several of the potential participants being grilled by men in the social group after the research screening interview. On two occasions, the interviewees were socially isolated after offering their explanations of their contact with the researchers. One additional individual had been pushed to the ground during an angry interchange. While the project's interpreter was not able to overhear everything that was said during the angry interchange, the upshot was significant anger surrounding contact with the Americans.

The meeting ended when co-PI Johnny Dietrich asked the committee to meet that evening and devise a consensus proposal for how to move forward with the project. Despite frustrated objections by the product development representative, the group decided on a plan to send an advance team to the refugee camps to discuss proper incentives with any available elders and/or consensus representatives of the camp population before finalizing the incentive package offered. One of the possibilities bandied about would involve augmenting the UN health care initiatives already available at the camps, so that the benefits would be spread more effectively across residents of the camps. The monetary amount would also be decided by the advance team, depending on the target value allowing the greatest cross-section of qualified camp residents to participate, while reducing risk of reprisals. Finally, elders would be asked to provide accurate communication to the camp residents regarding their credible support for assisting those with amputation injuries to overcome one of the pain-related disadvantages of their injuries.

Commentary

Researchers may propose to work with specific populations or in settings in which the consequences of such work may not be apparent without understanding the cultural context. In this case, proceeding with the research based on the proposed incentives without sensitivity to the population of interest increased the risk of harm to those participants. This clearly goes against both one's ethical obligations to respect other cultures and to prevent use of inappropriate research inducements in soliciting consent (Ethics Standards 8.02 and 8.06). In one sense, this case reflects positive and negative utilitarian consequences at odds (needed medical care versus social ostracism based on undue influence of incentives). Clearly, the moral rehabilitation psychologist would not knowingly participate in a project for which direct harm is a substantial risk and for which safeguards are not instituted. This type of decision reflects the intersection of nonmaleficence and respect for people's rights with the principle of justice and undue influence to achieve participation because of access to specific protocols or products.

This case highlights the issues surrounding (1) calculation of payment and its subsequent influence on consent, and (2) calculation of risk. Recent research has suggested that increased monetary incentives do not unduly influence study participants to consent to risks they might not otherwise accept (Halpern, Karlawish, Casarett, Berlin & Asch, 2004; Singer & Couper, 2008). In other words, incentives do not alter a person's assessment of a study's risks, even though the incentives can affect a person's willingness to participate. While these studies suggest that payments may not be coercive in soliciting consent, this is still a matter of debate given both studies involved hypothetical vignettes and only one (Halpern et al.) included medical risk. It also leaves open the question regarding how fair payment is determined. Sieber (2012) discusses four different models originally proposed by Ripley for determining fair payment to participants. These include market rate (based on supply and demand; used when recruitment criteria may be challenging to meet), wage rate (based on unskilled labor wage), reimbursement (cost neutral to participant), and fair share (community sharing). The author suggests that the wage model is "respectful of the needs of the poor" (p. 377), and the fair share model may be most appropriate when "an equitable relationship between the investigator and participating members of the community is viewed as very important" (p. 377). Both of these would be worth exploring, depending on study priorities.

The second issue is the researchers' ability to predict risks to participants. If the research team miscalculates the risks of participation, then justice is not served and harm may be a consequence. Making a rapid decision rather than a thoughtful one increases the risk of miscalculation of both influences and consequences. In this case, ethically responsible behavior necessitates further review of the psychologist's concerns prior to it even being possible to achieve informed consent, because both the stipends and the medical care can exert influences on decision-making with potentially disastrous results.

Although consequences may be unintended, they are not necessarily unpredictable. Researchers have a moral obligation to minimize risks that are potentially preventable. In addition, psychologists have a particular responsibility to protect those participating in research who are more vulnerable (vulnerability in this case created by medical and financial circumstances). The discussion turns around the concepts of undue inducement and undue profit (Emanuel, 2004; US Code of Federal Regulations, 2003) when conducting scientific research with populations that are comparatively economically disadvantaged when considering other social groups. To help cope with issues of vulnerability, the research team has to evaluate and ensure the "fairness" of the deal being made and its influence on the benefits and risks. Then, potential participants can make a more informed choice regarding participation.

Ultimately, one's moral responsibilities encompass both intentions and preventable (foreseeable) consequences. The research enterprise simply cannot work if researchers ignore the sensitivities of vulnerable populations. In this case, the refugee camps, not just the research participants selected out of those special populations, needed to value the work involved and, as such, were part of the solution.

Disposition

The study was ultimately completed within a few weeks of the original time frame, which grudgingly satisfied MegaMed. However, the amount of the individual monetary incentives increased by 36%, and the cost for providing an enhanced medical benefit to a broader group of camp residents increased significantly, bitter pills for the sponsoring medical equipment company to swallow. Nonetheless, the company was quick to sign off on the increased costs of those services in order to address their goal of manufacturing and selling an effective product.

Learning Opportunities

1. Research with underserved populations (often economically disadvantaged) can sometimes involve creating a contingency for participation that is difficult to refuse for someone without access to health care, or difficult to opt out of once risks are adequately explained. For some, health care research projects present the only mechanism of access to any health care services available to underserved populations. Design some safeguards that might be added to a research proposal to address these ethical concerns.
2. Evaluate the following statements in light of your own personal and social values, arriving at a conclusion that would satisfy a relative with whom you have a reciprocal relationship. *Illness is just bad luck. Some people have luck and others don't. Why should we have to contribute to a health care system that treats the unlucky?*

Brief Scenario: Dr. Goran Talcic had a wide smile on his face as he greeted his old friend Dr. Mike Mincey at the door to his splendid office suite. Both men had shared the rigors of preparation for and taking the ABPP examination in rehabilitation psychology several years earlier. They'd had time to share their career aspirations during their collaborative study sessions, each describing a very different mission on which each would embark once they had passed muster in the specialty. Success had shone on them after the exam, but Mike's career pathway had taken a stratospheric trajectory when compared to the inpatient rehabilitation team consultancy that Goran had undertaken. Given his broad-spectrum awareness of the staffing requirements of rehabilitation organizations, Mike (a retreaded computer engineer) had decided to create an employment hub that placed critical, high quality clinical rehabilitation staff in client venues around the country for a percentage of annual salaries. Mike had named the company Rehab PsyScreen, Inc.

Mike had experienced remarkable early success, with an 89% success rate (defined as retention at one year) with placement candidates across all disciplines during the first 2 years of operation. Aware of the variability in rehabilitation staff characters, working conditions, organizational structures, and performance expectations, Goran was more than impressed. He was eager to witness the details of the selection and placement process because Mike had recently offered him a position with his growing company. Smiling smugly, Mike led his friend to a security-locked door and pressed a complex combination. Before entering the room, Mike announced to Goran that what he was about to view was strictly proprietary. When the door opened, they entered a noticeably chilly controlled environment overrun by mega-computer hardware. Mike explained that what Goran was now privy to was his "nerve center," where electronic vetting of each placement candidate took place. Through carefully selected and politically connected friends, he had secured legal access to multiple pertinent health care and academic databases; state and federal regulatory, financial, and law enforcement agency archives (not requiring special national security clearance); and social media websites; he even had a few staffers employed solely to surf the web for new social media information pertinent to any of their burgeoning pool of job placement candidates. Mike proudly announced that not the slightest character flaw, error in social judgment, or performance misstep was allowed to pass muster in his pool of placement candidates. Goran, privately shocked at this revelation, initially thought back to the disturbing premise of the movie Gattaca—genetically honed "perfect" individuals screened and trained to serve in the astronaut corps; a screening scheme that invited challenge from motivationally driven, but "imperfect" talented individuals. He then contrasted this image with thoughts of the incredible potential of technology—being able to deliver rehabilitation expertise to underserved populations across the globe.

Brief Commentary: In this scenario the reader, taking on the character of Goran, must ask several important questions regarding the ethical nature of the business model adopted by his friend and fellow rehabilitation psychologist. First, the nature of **privacy and confidentiality** protections well established in both professional health care discipline protocols and in varied state legislation appear to raise cautions about invasion of personal privacy boundaries during screening processes. Related to these concerns, the current practice of some businesses accessing social media websites for information relevant to employees and job candidates are being challenged in the courts, claiming invasion of privacy. Second, it is unknown whether the selection criteria differentially affect individuals with disabilities and individuals carrying social or economic minority status. **Discrimination** on the basis of such factors is expressly discouraged in the Ethics Code, as well as being a violation of federal civil liberties law. Such a vetting process as described in the scenario cannot be automatically condemned as unduly biased without explanations of the above concerns.

Another area of concern is **informed consent** of both the candidates subject to microscopic character investigation, and organizations who sign on to receive those candidate employees who have survived the screening process. For example, in submitting an application, has each candidate provided tacit acceptance of the screening procedure? If the screening practice is cleared legally, would Goran's support of this practice be consistent with ethical behavior? Several questions related to screening come to mind in aspiring to uphold moral behavior. Does each constituency have adequate and sufficient knowledge of the details of the screening process in order to consent to participation? Have all of their questions regarding the degree of invasiveness of the screening been accurately and completely answered, or does the proprietary nature of the process require vague descriptions at times? Are such informational restrictions on **disclosure** accurately described by the company? Can these two constituencies make adequate decisions to participate or refuse participation in the placement service based on reasonably accurate knowledge to allow valid weighing of **costs and benefits**?

Simply because sophisticated technology exists, we should not be compelled toward its unmitigated use. Utilizing an ethics-based conceptual foundation to evaluate the values-based worth and proper application of technology can provide the health care professional of any ilk with a starting point in the struggle to grasp the implications of technology use across varied situations. We can use the legal system to address perceived injustices in application of technology. However, in many respects the legal system is reactionary, an evolutionary process of decisional refinements across time sparked by legal reactions and judgmental precedents. Relying solely on the legal system for answers sometimes requires that society endure **inequity** in policy application, and await corrective legal action before an on-balance solution is discovered. The effective utilization of ethical conceptualization, an accretion and distillation of knowledge from centuries of philosophical thought and validated against the results of countless instances of social contextual application of and experience with these concepts, facilitates planning and problem-solving prior to action.

RELEVANT STANDARDS

1.02 Conflicts between Ethics and Law, Regulations, or Other Governing Legal Authority
1.04 Informal Resolution of Ethical Violations
3.01 Unfair Discrimination
3.04 Avoiding Harm
3.06 Conflict of Interest
4.02 Discussing Limits of Confidentiality
4.04 Minimizing Intrusions on Privacy
4.05 (a, b) Disclosures
4.07 (2, 3) Use of Confidential Information for Didactic or Other Purposes

6 Principle: Respect for People's Rights and Dignity

TAKING A CUE from the APA Ethics Code, this principle is defined as awareness of and safeguarding the rights and dignity of persons served by rehabilitation psychologists, with a focus on privacy, confidentiality, and self-determination. While privacy laws vary significantly across states, rules and regulations surrounding confidentiality (with the passage of HIPAA) have been homogeneously spread across all health care organizations receiving federal health insurance monies (Medicare and Medicaid) for services rendered. Self-determination, on the other hand, is a universal ethical concept most closely linked to the bioethical principle of respect for autonomy (Beauchamp & Childress, 2009). While Beauchamp and Childress are reluctant to state that respect for autonomy is an overarching bioethics principle, it certainly is the principle with the most legal precedent and legislation supporting its basic tenets. The primary applied ethics concept related to the principle of autonomy is the process of informed consent. For example, *Canterbury vs. Spence* (1972) is a classic case establishing the patient's right to receive reasonable information on which to base health care decisions. (In this case, a 19-year-old underwent a laminectomy for back pain and fell postoperatively, resulting in additional surgery and multiple complications. Dr. Spence was sued for failure to inform the patient of the potential risks and alternative treatments.) The fundamental concepts underlying the APA Ethics Code (APA, 2002) principle of respect for people's rights and dignity are the protection and preservation of a person's right to choose what happens to them and their personal information in the context of health care service provision.

In rehabilitation, psychologists commonly must balance right to privacy with beneficence and nonmaleficence (i.e., do no harm) because of the patient populations served. Sound judgment about the patient's ability (i.e., competence) to engage in informed decision-making is critical to ethical practice and is faced directly and perhaps most frequently in individuals with severe cognitive impairment. While paternalistic decision-making very early in patient recovery (e.g., emergence from coma) may be justifiable, the water can become murkier as patient recovery progresses. The psychologist needs to determine the circumstances that reasonably dictate a shift from surrogate decision-making to patient decision-making. As patients are increasingly able to consistently and reliably communicate their preferences in specific situations, the psychologist has an ethical obligation to discern when the patient has achieved the capacity to give informed consent; this represents a fundamental application of the principle of respect for autonomy.

Establishing a patient's capacity to give informed consent typically assumes some level of shared information-processing. This allows the psychologist to determine whether the patient has a reasonable understanding of critical information and can manipulate that information (i.e., rationally weigh pros and cons and likely consequences) in such a way as to express an uncoerced, reliable preference or choice. (See Hanson & Kerkhoff, 2004, for a detailed discussion of soliciting consent from individuals with compromised cognitive function.) Informed consent also assumes a certain level of good occurring at various points in the rehabilitation process. First, the patient minimally acquires a basic understanding of the issues involved in rehabilitation decisions, which (at least theoretically) may facilitate realistic expectations for intervention. Second, creating a dialogue around informed consent fosters the development of a trusting relationship. Third, the patient and/or family can begin thinking about how to plan for potential future needs. Fourth, the patient may be more willing to engage in specific services because the groundwork for those services has been laid. Finally, informed consent discussions provide the rehabilitation psychologist with a window of understanding into both the patient's decisional capacity and the family's current emotional status and coping reserves based on their reactions to questions asked.

Of course, initiating this process creates some risk of negative consequences. For example, despite being capable of making a decision, the patient may not do so based on the gravity of the situation or perceived pressure inadvertently created by the decision-making process. This occurs especially in individuals with compromised coping skills resulting from cognitive or emotional decline or unresolved family issues that shift decision-making authority away from the patient. The end result could be even poorer coping because of premature consideration of issues the patient or family is not yet ready to manage. Cultural factors, especially when family structure varies from Western traditions, may influence how informed consent approaches are received. Decisions are not without consequences, and the ability to consider potential consequences is not the same as responding to them when one has been the decision-maker who contributes to a specific outcome. When the decision-maker is already coping with a catastrophic injury or chronic illness, it may be particularly difficult to anticipate the impact of specific decisions, and this challenges tentative defenses and reserves. This latter point will be illustrated in our first case example.

> CASE EXAMPLE 6.1
>
> "I just want to get outta here...!"

I. Quick Reference

Critical Incident

A rehabilitation psychologist who is licensed, but whose primary role is administrative, is asked by a colleague to intervene with Moses Reed, a patient who is refusing medical treatment and wants to be discharged. Mr. Reed has endured several unsuccessful attempts to insert a gastric feeding tube secondary to edema-related dysphagia. Only local anesthesia was employed during the most recent attempt, which resulted in an emotionally traumatized gentleman who does not want to repeat the experience, despite an urgent need to achieve a patent pathway for nutrition. The nasogastric tube that he was left with is beginning to erode his throat tissue and should be removed. The patient is understandably distressed by these repeated medical procedures. However, his treatment refusal and the request to be discharged have the potential to cause the patient grave harm. The patient's level of understanding of the current problem and consequences of leaving the rehabilitation hospital against medical advice are directly affected by his strong emotional reaction to the failed procedures. Additionally, his distressed emotional state makes soliciting adequately informed consent difficult. That said, decision-making capacity for basic health-related concepts is judged to be adequate in this case.

In the atypical role of administrator, the rehabilitation psychologist, Dr. Ministratore, must seek a solution that will protect this patient from potentially dire risk should he return home without the G-tube insertion procedure. If you were the psychologist, what would you need to consider in fulfilling your ethical obligations to this patient and to the health care organization? Use the following questions as guides.

- What are the components required to achieve minimally acceptable standards for determining informed consent?
- How would you approach the consent process with an individual whose emotional stability is precarious?

- Under what circumstances would you override the patient's right to refuse treatment?
- Are there any circumstances under which a "best interests" standard of surrogate decision-making would be more appropriate than substituted judgment?
- Under what circumstances would a health care organization's rights take precedence over a patient's rights?

Resolution

A. ***Patient is discharged against medical advice (AMA) without clinical follow-up but with referral to Adult Protective Services***

    Pro
    a) *Directly honors patient stated preferences (e.g., right to refuse care)*

    Con
    a) *Knowingly places patient at significant health risk*
    b) *Potential for incomplete understanding of consequences related to AMA discharge*
    c) *Burden placed on unprepared family for patient care and protection*
    d) *No accommodations for community transition, creating safety risks*
    e) *Adult Protective Services protections likely perceived as punitive*

B. ***Patient is discharged against medical advice with accommodations***

    Pro
    a) *Honors patient stated preferences (right to refuse); no guarantee of adequate understanding*
    b) *Provides protections via community transition accommodations; including APS education/rationale*

    Con
    a) *Knowingly places patient at significant health risk; potentially preventable*
    b) *Burden for care and safety placed on family and social agency; realistic prediction of substantial risk*
    c) *Unmet patient needs regarding nutrition and potential respiratory compromise*

C. ***Engage patient in informed consent process and determine informed decision***

    Pro
    a) *Honors patient preferences with adequate understanding of predictable risks*

TABLE 6.1
CASE ANALYSIS SUMMARY

Ethical Principles	Relevant Standards	Context & Key Stakeholders	Organizational & Legal Issues	Alternative Solutions
I. Primary Respect for People's Rights and Dignity - The clinicians and the administration of the rehab center must respect the patient's right to refuse treatment and discharge against medical advice, without applying coercion II. Secondary Beneficence & Nonmaleficence - The rehab center must advocate for patient safety and reduce risk of harm from decisions made Integrity - The RP must carefully delineate both clinical and administrative roles and responsibilities attendant to each role when addressing the patient	2.04 Bases for Scientific and Professional Judgment - The RP must adhere to scientific/ clinical data in presenting information to the patient 3.04 Avoiding Harm - The RP must be proactive in reducing the risk of harm to the patient 3.09 Cooperation with other Professionals - The RP must integrate his dual roles of clinician and administrator to the benefit of the patients and the program 3.10 Informed Consent - The RP must endeavor to adequately inform the patient regarding the health care risks and benefits of the proposed treatment	Patient – is faced with both an emotional and data-based decision RP—plays dual roles ARNP – program director who is advocating for her patient Elder Sister - Advocating for the emotional and physical needs of her brother GI Team - Willing to provide anesthesia for the next procedure Rehab Center - Advocating for the safety, legal rights, and benefit of their patient	Organizational Policy & Procedure - Provisions for patients to make decisions, choose treatment, and refuse treatment from an informed perspective State law - Establishing and protecting the patient's legal right to refuse treatment and to discharge from health care facilities against medical advice; must be informed of consequences of the latter	A. The patient discharges against medical advice; deny all postdischarge accommodations; recommend Adult Protective Services B. The patient discharges against medical advice; provide reasonable accommodations C. Adequately inform patient about risks and benefits of his right to choose and refuse treatment D. Adequately inform patient about risks and benefits of his right to choose and refuse treatment; encourage the preferred treatments without coercion via information and family input E. Seek court-mandated treatment to prevent poor physical outcome

b) *Community accommodations/protections offered with rationale provided*

Con

a) *Knowingly places patient at significant health risk; potentially preventable*
b) *Care/safety burden on family and social agency; realistic prediction of substantial risk*
c) *Remains at risk regarding nutrition and respiratory compromise*

D. **Engage patient in informed consent process and encourage treatment—Preferred**

Pro

a) *Honors patient right to choose/refuse treatment with adequate understanding of consequences; with rationale for community protections, if required*
b) *Safeguards against coercion in process of adequately informing patient and family*
c) *Places family in position of adaptive influence, given stated motivation for patient safety*
d) *Increases chances of adaptive choice for treatment to reduce health risk*

Con

a) *Chance of treatment refusal remains; but validated in the face of adequate understanding of risks/consequences*

E. **Seek court order to reinitiate treatment against patient's wishes**

Pro

a) *Treatment to preserve health provided, resulting in positive physical health outcome based on application of a best interests standard of decision-making*
b) *Team serves their perceived best long-term interests of patient*
c) *Long-term benefit of improved physical health likely stabilizes emotionality and therefore outweighs short-term harm*

Con

a) *Paternalistic approach jeopardizes trust and any future relationship with health care organization*
b) *Coping could rapidly deteriorate*
c) *Patient refusal could be played out in poor follow-up self-care, wasting time and resources*

II. Contextual Influences

Moses Reed is a 46-year-old African American gentleman who had experienced increasing weakness in his arms and legs over the previous seven months. Moses was never a person to run to the medical clinic unless he felt that he was at death's door. However, after repeated urgings from his family and his family physician (whom he implicitly trusted across many years of personal care), Moses finally agreed to a diagnostic workup. When a severe cervical stenosis with spinal cord impingement was discovered, surgery was recommended as the only viable treatment to preserve his neurological function.

Although the complex surgery proceeded flawlessly, on post-op day two, postsurgical edema compressed the cranial nerves and structures controlling Moses's swallowing reflex, such that he was unable to take in any nutrition by mouth. Both the family physician and the neurosurgery treatment team managed to convince Moses that he needed a nasogastric (NG) feeding tube, which was placed with some difficulty. This method of nutrition was barely tolerable to Moses, but he was reassured the tube would be temporary.

When the hoped-for quick resolution to the swallowing problem did not occur, the Gastro Intestinal (GI) lab tried several nonsedated, swallow-assisted approaches to insert a fiber optic tube into his stomach for inspection and probable gastric feeding tube (G-tube) placement. However, the fiber optic tube used to guide the G-tube placement could not pass the swollen portion of Moses' throat, and Moses was emotionally traumatized by the repeated attempts, finally refusing further efforts.

The next day, Moses was discharged, NG tube still in place, to the rehabilitation center. Distraught about his perceived maltreatment in the acute hospital, Moses demanded to be sent home during his initial rehabilitation center evaluation. Prior to Moses's departure from the acute hospital, his family physician and the nursing team had informed Moses about the risky consequences of his desire to immediately return home before his nutritional status was stabilized and functional everyday living abilities improved. The NG tube could only be in place for a short while because of the risk of throat tissue erosion—evidence of which had already begun to emerge. The only other option for nutrition was a central feeding line—no one's optimal choice in this case. Those concerns triggered the medical team's decision to send Moses to the inpatient rehabilitation center under medical care and observation, instead of directly home.

Dr. Eduardo Ministratore, trained as a rehabilitation psychologist and then a health administrator, was the chief operating officer of the South Inlet Rehabilitation Center where Moses Reed was admitted. Dr. Ministratore was approached by Mary Joyner, ARNP, a colleague and program manager of the new spinal cord injury unit, to intervene with Mr. Reed. Apparently, the psychologist serving that unit was absent, and coverage was not available in a timely manner. The rehabilitation psychologist proposed an initial conversation with the patient, accompanied by Mary

Joyner, with whom the patient had formed basic rapport. Dr. Ministratore's primary responsibilities in this situation were to attempt to adequately inform the patient regarding the risk-reducing treatment, and to serve the primary mission of the rehabilitation facility, which was to provide safe, high quality treatment to everyone admitted.

While communicative during the initial interview, it became obvious that Moses Reed was not a person who easily accepted either evaluation or intervention from the health care system. In fact, he was quite suspicious of the technology that suffused the health care system, feeling that "those infernal machines" stood firmly between patients and their health care providers, impeding the development of trust in the care relationship. He simply wanted to return home and resume his life routine. After the pertinent information was communicated and patient comprehension evidenced, Moses was left to consider the detailed recommendation of the rehabilitation team to consent to the G-tube placement.

After this conversation, Dr. Ministratore and Mary Joyner conferred. They decided that other individuals who were influential in Mr. Reed's life needed to be involved in the conversation, especially the family. A second consideration was to involve the family practitioner, as a trusted health care professional. However, staging the supporting cast in serial fashion would likely present a less threatening scenario to the patient. Moses's family was the first to be contacted.

Upon hearing about their brother's request to leave the rehabilitation center, Mr. Reed's siblings' initial response was to supportively advocate for his return home. However, they reversed their stance once they realized that he was very likely going to extubate himself once home. They were also concerned about being unable to physically assist him in his weakened neurological condition. Mr. Reed's elder sister agreed to intervene with her brother in the decision-making process.

During a follow-up conversation among Mr. Reed, Ed Ministratore, Mary Joyner and Moses's elder sister geared to inform him of the critical details of the proposed procedure, a strategy emerged that posed a potential resolution. By offering the patient general anesthesia, utilizing Propofol—an anesthetic agent that relaxed the muscles of the throat—the fiber optic tube to help illuminate and guide the G-tube placement could be inserted more easily than in the past attempts. Not being awake and aware during the procedure held a certain appeal for Mr. Reed, who did not argue with the basic goal of having proper nutrition in order to facilitate recovery and return home. He also acknowledged the caregiving needs of his family. His current weakened state would only force his family to "pester me all the more to behave." In the company of his sister, and after a brief phone call with his family physician who supported the procedure, Moses finally agreed to the recommendation proposed by the health care team.

Commentary

Based on supportive legal precedent and regulatory changes in health care, informed consent has evolved from a passive to an active process. For example, simply obtaining a signature on a consent form is no longer sufficient because it does not confirm patient understanding of the variables influencing any decision reached. Rather, the psychologist needs to engage the patient in discussing the potential implications of decisions and must be reasonably certain the patient is making an informed, uncoerced choice. But what does the patient need to understand? Multiple components of the APA Ethics Code provide very limited guidance regarding what psychologists must cover when soliciting informed consent. For example, the 2002 revised Code includes a general informed consent standard (ES 3.10) as well as specific standards applicable to assessment (ES 9.03), treatment (ES 10.0), and research (ES 8.02). That said, these standards provide only minimal information regarding the content elements of consent. Generally speaking, consent must involve adequate coverage of the problem in comprehensible language so that the patient understands the specific issue and associated risks and benefits of the care being recommended. If the patient's understanding of the issues can be confirmed, then soliciting an uncoerced decision from the patient can proceed. If patient understanding is not evident across assessments (e.g., via the patient recapping material in his own words or other assessment strategy), a surrogate decision will be required.

Communicating what patients should reasonably understand is a challenge rehabilitation psychologists commonly face, given the various impediments that are part and parcel of many diagnoses necessitating rehabilitation admission. In the case of Mr. Reed, his coping issues were negatively affecting his ability to exercise a reasoned, deliberative approach to evaluating his need for further care. Therefore, the psychologist prioritized actions initially to address the emotional factors hindering the patient's processing. By using a nonthreatening, sequential approach to information provision and partnering with the only people the patient appeared to trust on any level (Mary Joyner, his sister, his family physician), the psychologist was able to constructively mitigate the impact of the patient's emotional reactivity on the decision being made. If this had not occurred, legal counsel might have been necessary regarding steps to protect both the patient and the organization, depending on the outcome of the determination of the patient's capacity to make a decision in this circumstance. The greater the risk of harm to the patient, the more advisable it is to seek counsel. The state's interest can become more compelling as the gravity of the consequences (defined as the ability to reverse an outcome) increases. Regardless of current law and regulatory mandates, one needs look no further than the Schiavo case in Florida to appreciate the complexity of adhering to respect for patient or surrogate rights, when the predictability of outcome and/or the clarity of communication regarding present health status and associated decisions are questioned (*Bush v. Schiavo*, 2004; Quill, 2005; *Schindler Schiavo v. Schiavo*, 2005).

In the present case, there is no mention of the procedure used to determine Mr. Reed's comprehension of the implications of being discharged home or his ultimate decision to stay (see "Disposition" below). Whether or not a patient concurs with the health care provider's recommendations should not determine whether the patient's decision is accepted; competent individuals are entitled to make decisions that others may judge unwise or even unsafe. The psychologist made a reasonable assumption that the patient's immediate prior experience, combined with his history of suspiciousness toward the health care system, resulted in the emotional reactivity leading to treatment refusal. However, the psychologist failed to evaluate the emotional drivers behind the patient's change of heart and therefore only partially fulfilled his ethical obligations regarding adequate consent based on the information presented.

Finally, in this instance, the administrator-psychologist acted simultaneously on behalf of the patient and the organization. Therefore, Dr. Ministratore's dual roles as a licensed rehabilitation psychologist and administrator were complementary. While the patient rights advocate role is a familiar one for the rehabilitation psychologist, the management role is less commonly filled by members of the specialty, but is no less valid vis-à-vis an individual patient in need. The health care organization has an ethical vested interest in preserving patient safety (Weber, 2001). To this end, the psychologist fulfilled both advocacy roles, given that he could validly and simultaneously advocate for the patient's decisional autonomy and the organization's mission of providing quality care in a safe environment without compromising ethical principles in either role.

Disposition

Moses Reed ultimately decided to proceed with the G-tube placement. The tipping point during the decision-making conversation was reached when his sister reminded Moses that she just could not bear his coming to harm at home. She emphasized the point by "threatening" to move in with him because she would not be able to sleep in her own house, knowing that he was "slowly starving to death."

The next morning, the procedure went well—without complications. After returning to South Inlet Rehab Center, Mr. Reed was increasingly able to focus his renewed physical and emotional energies on gaining strength and functional skills through rehabilitation treatment. He returned home after several weeks, with the G-tube still in place. The fact that he was able to begin oral nutrition—under the watchful eye of the rehabilitation program's speech language pathologist while still an inpatient—enabled him to gain increasing pleasure from eating... despite the fact that his fare was hospital food. He actually expressed an eagerness to return home to his own home cooking—canned goods flavored with hot sauce.

Moses was able to have the G-tube removed 6 weeks after placement, again without incident. By that time, he had graduated from Home Health Care therapies to outpatient rehabilitation treatment, having returned to modified independent living.

Learning Opportunities

1. Under what circumstances would you deem it advisable to consult legal counsel regarding patient decision-making?
2. List several strategies that you might or do employ to increase the patient's active role in health care decision-making in your work environment.
3. Under what circumstances would you seek the counsel of a patient's designated surrogate in making health care decisions?

Brief Scenario: Celeste Stemple, a 16-year-old patient in the hematology unit, was referred to the Psychology Department's Consultation and Liaison service for evaluation of a possible anxiety disorder. As a rehabilitation psychologist by training, you seek to involve the patient's mother in the evaluative process. Her mother, Hilary, has been routinely visiting her daughter throughout her hospitalization and has made it known to staff that she is to be involved with all treatment decisions in the course of protecting her minor child. During the preparation phase of the evaluation, you note in the medical record that Celeste is HIV+ (via vertical transmission from mother in utero). Further discussion with the patient's mother reveals that Celeste is not aware of her diagnosis. Her mother had prevented her from knowing about the diagnosis, having explained to Celeste that the medication they both take as far back as she can remember is treatment for an immune system disorder that they share. Celeste has never questioned her mother in this regard. Further, Mrs. Stemple is adamant about keeping this information from her daughter until she determines that the "time is right." However, she is unable to provide any criteria for that determination. How would you address this potentially significant challenge, given that Celeste might inadvertently transmit her viral infection to another person? What are the rights of adolescents regarding access to their health care information? What factors affect potential access? What are the ethical issues at odds in determining next steps?

Brief Commentary: The scenario reminds us of the varied health care settings in which rehabilitation psychologists, by virtue of their extensive training in the team treatment model, provide psychological services. In this case, Celeste is a minor whose legal **decision-making rights** are held by her mother Hilary. The rehabilitation psychologist is faced with evaluating and treating a teenaged patient who presents with anxiety of unknown duration and etiology. Review of the EMR reveals a "family secret" of her HIV infection, the potential for sexual behavior that presents an unintentional transmission risk, and her mother's emotional status regarding her own HIV infection and parental responsibility for vertical transmission to her child. Needless to say, the case presents a complex set of challenges to the consultation.

The rehabilitation psychologist must first focus on the needs of his patient in determining the root of her anxiety, in the context of her current hematology unit admission. Depending on the patient's understanding of her current health status, the anxiety may be directly or indirectly linked to her medical history and the unknowns enforced by her mother. While the adolescent cannot formally consent to medical treatment, she is certainly in a position to **assent** to such treatment. From the behavioral perspective, assent provides the minor child with the rationale for treatment, so that commitment to the treatment process can be properly reinforced. Therefore, assent requires that Celeste receive disclosure of pertinent facts related to her treatment, including underlying condition, the plan of care, prognosis, treatment alternatives, and benefits/costs associated with all treatment choices available.

The Ethics Code presents the rehabilitation psychologist with ample support for discussing the timing of informing her daughter with the mother; as Celeste matures, the risk of inadvertent transmission of her HIV infection increases—highlighting a social responsibility to **protect society from a preventable harm**. Honoring Celeste's moral right to participate in decision-making regarding her own health from an informed position can be the focal point of a conversation between the psychologist and mother. If successful, a follow-up conversation among the patient, her mother and rehabilitation psychologist (in a supportive role) can occur that begins to explore the implications of their HIV infections. In addition, state law may mandate disclosure of HIV infection to a sexual partner (via the health department or physician or individual). Therefore, partner notification requirements may provide another avenue for discussion given the teen's developmental level.

RELEVANT ETHICS STANDARDS
3.04 Avoiding Harm
3/10 (2, 4) Informed Consent
4.05 (a, b 3) Disclosures

> CASE EXAMPLE 6.2
>
> "Didn't you hear me say NO…!"

I. Quick Reference
Critical Incident

Dr. Megan Morrissey began her workday at St. Alphonso Rehabilitation Hospital in the usual manner by checking the electronic health record for new admissions and referrals to the Rehabilitation Psychology Service. She identified a new patient, one Pete Snodgrass. His history revealed that Pete had sustained compound fractures in three extremities (each with non-weight-bearing restrictions) in a work-related injury. Management of pain was apparently a major challenge in the case. Fortunately, there was no evidence of a brain injury. While having sustained this major multitrauma did not distinguish him from Pete's fellow patients, his behavior certainly did.

From the moment Mr. Snodgrass entered the rehabilitation center, his bad temper, worse language, and limited willingness to cooperate in the admission process had endeared him to no one among the staff. His medical status might have engendered sympathetic support from the rehabilitation team members had his behavior not alienated potential helpers.

Armed with official medical and unofficial staff opinion data, Dr. Morrissey went to evaluate her new patient. When she entered the room, Pete Snodgrass was lying in bed in a contorted manner that simply could not be comfortable, sheet pulled up over his head. As soon as she introduced herself, Dr. Morrissey received a flat refusal from the patient regarding any contact with a mental health professional. Despite her best efforts to win over the recalcitrant gentleman, he would not budge from his position of rejecting her services. She left the room in a quandary.

If you were the rehabilitation psychologist and have been called on to help the team intervene with this patient, what would you consider appropriate next steps? Consider the following questions in making your decisions.

- Given the patient's history, are there any direct steps you could take to engage him in providing psychological services?
    - If yes, how would you approach the patient?
    - If no, on what do you base this decision, and how confident are you that the patient's initial negative reaction reflects his true convictions, given his challenging physical limitations and painful discomfort caused by trauma?

TABLE 6.2
CASE ANALYSIS SUMMARY

Ethical Principles	Relevant Standards	Context & Key Stakeholders	Organizational & Legal Issues	Alternative Solutions
I. Primary Respect for People's Rights and Dignity - The patient has the right to refuse treatment; however, the needs of the patient must be considered in the rehabilitation context regarding safety and risk of harm II. Secondary Beneficence & Nonmaleficence - The RP must endeavor to reduce risk of harm and advocate for benefit, even if providing for the patient indirectly; The RP must also weigh the patient's behavior in context of disruption to the broader rehab environment Fidelity & Responsibility - The RP must provide for the safety of team members and viability of the rehab program for this patient as part of her role on the team	3.04 Avoiding harm—The RP must provide safeguards, albeit indirectly, to prevent avoidable AMA discharge 3.09 Cooperation with other professionals - An RP role on the team is to help integrate services 3.05 Multiple relationships— The RP is tasked with multiple roles and relationships on the team, providing opportunities to positively impact patient program performance in different ways 3.10 Informed Consent—The RP abides by patient refusal in terms of direct intervention; but addresses needs indirectly	Patient - refuses RP treatment; has psychological intervention needs RP—Respects patient treatment refusal and provides team guidance to manage the patient's behavior Rehab Team - Varied professionals manage patient behavior and outcome via collaboration with RP and each other Rehab Hospital - Allows indirect behavioral intervention on behalf of patient and staff to ensure safety and quality care	Organization's Policy & Procedure - Demands informed consent for treatment; permits flexible provision of behavioral management services outside direct treatment arrangement; broader admissions policy and impact on types of patients admitted warrants consideration related to team training; consultation on team is part of rehabilitation milieu and overall consenting process State law - Legal right to refuse treatment; informed consent to treat; requires patient understanding of consequences of decisions regarding treatment refusal and ability to communicate that understanding	A. Honor treatment refusal and drop case involvement B. Honor treatment refusal for direct treatment but continue to advise the team in the patient's best interests C. Ignore treatment refusal, considering such a decision ill-informed, and continue to provide direct services D. Transfer to another facility with more structured behavioral management

- Does intentional indirect influence of rehabilitation team treatment and care violate the patient's right of choice? Why or why not?

Resolutions

   A. ***Honor treatment refusal and offer no further services***
                        Pro
      a) *Honors patient right to refuse treatment*
                        Con
      a) *Treatment needs ignored*
      b) *Patient's rehabilitation program effectiveness and efficiency compromised because of behavioral disruption without RP intervention*

   B. ***Honor patient's right to refuse treatment but advise team—Preferred***
                        Pro
      a) *Honors treatment refusal for direct intervention*
      b) *Provides for indirect adaptive behavior management via team implementation of behavior management guidelines generated by RP*
                        Con
      a) *Treatment more aligned with psychology provided instead by other team disciplines*
      b) *No clarification sought from the patient regarding indirect program involvement of the RP-consultative role; a strategic decision in patient's best interests*

   C. ***Ignore treatment refusal and continue to provide services***
                        Pro
      a) *Patient receives, albeit under duress, direct behavioral intervention*
                        Con
      a) *Any potential gains from behavioral intervention likely to be circumvented by patient distress regarding RP ignoring his right to refuse*
      b) *Could lead to valid legal challenge by patient*
      c) *Ignores Ethics Code standards regarding patient's right to refuse treatment*
      d) *Could lead to deterioration of patient's working relationship with other team members, compromising program gains*

   D. ***Transfer to another facility combining more structured behavioral management with rehabilitation***
                        Pro
      a) *Breaks negative cycle between team and patient*
      b) *New facility benefits from rehabilitation team experience to structure program*

Con

a) *Another facility may not be available within a reasonable distance and may not be funded*
b) *Given history, likely shifts challenges to another site rather than creating treatment plan to address internally*
c) *Informed consent for transfer may prove challenging*

II. Contextual Influences

Pete Snodgrass had lived a rough life during his 42 years. His family had disowned him when he was labeled "incorrigible" by the juvenile justice system at age 15. Pete had been in and out of various local jails and state prisons his whole life, mostly for unarmed robbery and drug possession, ultimately spending more time behind bars than in the community. Pete had no family or friends in the community. He was asleep in the rear of a truck, unbeknownst to the driver, when the heavy produce load the driver was carrying was dumped, along with Pete, who sustained crush injuries to both his legs and left arm and multiple rib fractures.

Dr. Megan Morrissey, on the other hand, had a very different life history. Her graduate and postgraduate training in rehabilitation psychology was a natural fit. Eleven years later, she was a seasoned professional and felt at home in the rehabilitation team milieu. She was of the opinion that 95% of the individuals she had encountered in her years of practice eventually bought into the team-based rehabilitation treatment model, no matter how rocky their introduction. Megan was determined to secure Pete's buy-in to the rehabilitation program, even if she had to do it at a distance.

Because Megan had not acquired Pete's permission for direct psychology services, she instead assisted the team in interacting with Pete in a psychologically informed and effective manner. She created behavioral management guidelines, posted in the EMR for ease of staff access. It was her hope that the concrete nature of activities of daily living (ADLs) and mobility tasks would appeal to Pete's practical view of the world and that he would view these rehabilitation activities as opportunities to return to the community, a point she emphasized with the staff.

Megan left open the option with Pete to work directly with her, and she continued to work with the team. As the team shared new behavioral observation data, Megan effectively modified the behavioral strategies to counter Pete's unacceptable behavioral manipulations. Second, when Pete intimidated fellow patients, Dr. Morrissey advised the team physiatrist to read Pete the riot act, such that a firm and nonnegotiable limit regarding lack of respect shown to fellow patients was set. Importantly, when Pete was hauled up short by the physician, he showed mild remorse. He explained that he had never intentionally disrespected fellow inmates if they had not deserved such behavior. Last, Dr. Morrissey consulted with the occupational therapist in charge of the outpatient work evaluation program. Dr. Morrissey described Mr. Snodgrass, including the objectionable behavior, but couched the challenging case in terms of a gentleman whose employment potential had never been tested.

Pete Snodgrass's care needs required that he be admitted to a subacute rehabilitation program nested within an extended care facility (ECF). While initially rebelling against this perceived indignity, the patient reluctantly admitted that he continued to need some assistance with ADLs and mobility, so agreed to the transfer. Meanwhile, Dr. Morrissey had anticipated that Mr. Snodgrass would eventually become bored with his long recuperation under non-weight-bearing restrictions, especially in the confines of the ECF. Once that occurred, Pete might be more tractable regarding proactive planning for outpatient treatment. She hoped that he would accept outpatient OT intervention, especially as the therapist's interventions related to vocational applications. Dr. Morrissey could then refer the patient to one of her colleagues in the State Department of Vocational Rehabilitation for assistance in finding job training.

Commentary

This case creates an interesting question regarding multiple relationships, given the psychologist had professional responsibilities to both the patient and the rehabilitation team, which was directly engaged with the patient. It is almost universally the case that psychologists working in rehabilitation settings have obligations to multiple parties. In this case, the patient was a potential consumer, but the team proved to be the primary provider of services, given that the patient declined psychological services. Patient treatment refusal does not prevent the psychologist from fulfilling her team responsibilities. Therefore, the psychologist needed to ensure appropriate boundaries in interacting with the team regarding the patient, consistent with the ethical principle of fidelity and responsibility.

That said, the psychologist may have been unduly influenced by the patient's history and initial presentation in making a quick judgment not to provide direct services based on the patient's choice to refuse such services. The psychologist formally interacted directly with the patient on only one occasion. Limits placed on inpatient rehabilitation stays can unfortunately but necessarily weigh on the approach that the psychologist adopts in order to facilitate greater patient independence. In this case, the psychologist may have had the opportunity to subtly and directly influence the patient's behavior by small, incremental interventions in the patient's room or in the treatment milieu. At a minimum, one has to ask whether the psychologist prematurely ruled out direct intervention, especially if one considers the variability of response and recovery from traumatic injury. *Informed consent is a process, not an event.* The process of informed consent reflects both the ongoing evaluation of a person's decisional capacity and the serial communication required to ensure adequate understanding—on their own terms—of the elements of any personal or health care decision. Is it possible that biases inadvertently influenced the psychologist's choice not to directly follow up with the patient?

The patient's social history and initial presentation provide meaningful evidence to understand the patient's behavior. This independent-minded patient was rendered a "fish out of water," who had experienced a dramatic role shift toward dependency. He lacked social assets outside of prison. With no family or friends available, he demonstrated poor interpersonal skills when expressing health care choices, and lacked coping skills for postdischarge planning that might improve his overall life's circumstances. All of these behaviors are considered high risk for treatment failure (Knapp & Gavazzi, 2012). These issues highlight the challenges this patient would have likely had forming productive relationships with the rehabilitation team even under nonstressful circumstances. However, the psychologist needs to consider these factors in evaluating her response to the patient's initial treatment refusal, and whether defined strategies to intervene with high risk patients (e.g., address treatment reluctance up front; enhanced vigilance regarding patient's needs, therapeutic boundaries, and potential threats to therapeutic alliance) would have made a difference (Knapp & Gavazzi, 2012).

Regardless of the outcome of the informed consent process, the indirect influence with the team is a sound independent or complementary approach to patient intervention. Dr. Morrissey elected to stay engaged with the patient via indirect influence developing behavioral management guidelines for the team to implement, coaching team members in preparation for limit-setting interactions with the patient, and involving team members whose treatment focus reinforced the patient's desire to return to viable employment. Therefore, the psychologist's influence with the team occurred on two levels. First, the psychologist applied her understanding of the patient's psychological characteristics to provide practical strategies for the team to interact effectively with the patient. Second, and perhaps equally importantly, the psychologist successfully assisted the team with their emotional reactivity to the patient by providing prompt, adaptive responses when the patient attempted to initiate disruptive actions or escalate conflict. The rehabilitation psychologist's success with the team directly influenced the team's ability to manage their emotional resources in response to this patient. Ultimately, this sets the stage for future responsiveness and effectiveness when patients present challenging behavior.

Another primary case issue is the patient's lack of funding. The economic perspective, especially as it may apply to a consultant contracted to an inpatient rehabilitation facility can be ethically troublesome. While rehabilitation psychologists are urged via the Ethics Code to provide pro bono services to those indigent individuals in need of treatment, treatment refusal by a patient referred for services is another matter. If a consultant is totally dependent on private direct service billing in order to maintain a contract, treatment refusal by a referred patient presents an ethically valid reason for not providing services. Such circumstances should be acknowledged in the contractual arrangement between the consultant and HCO. However, in this case example there is a contractual nuance. Dr. Morrissey's salary and benefit costs are partially offset by clinical billing (provided by the organization) for services. Contractually, the rehabilitation psychologist is expected to generate an explicit monthly percentage of salary and benefits costs via billing for services. Thus, the consultant must be aware of ongoing rates of direct service provision in order to fulfill this contractual requirement.

This consultancy contract also contains a codicil allowing "administrative costs" to be paid to the psychologist at an agreed on hourly rate—in addition to payments derived from direct patient service billing. Such professional activities might include team conference contributions, presenting in-services to the team, program development activities, and so forth. Therefore, we see the rehabilitation psychologist in this case exercising the explicit role of contributing team member—an organizationally valid role expectation detailed in the consultancy contract. It is in the contractual category of "administrative costs" that consultant contributions to team performance efficiency and effectiveness regarding individual patients in extraordinary circumstances. Obviously, this contractual benefit is to be exercised sparingly. Indeed, this case is atypical in that respect.

Disposition

Pete Snodgrass proved to be a willing client when it came time to take part in vocational programming. He, with the assistance of his rehabilitation case manager, had managed to locate a transitional living program for which he qualified while he completed his outpatient treatment. Though he did not finish high school, Pete had secured a GED while in prison. He proudly considered the preparatory work for the GED examination relatively easy, reluctantly admitting that he had wished at the time he could have gone further in school. Working with his assigned VR counselor, Pete agreed to apply for Social Security and state identification cards. While his felony history limited some of his legal rights, Pete was willing to attempt to access the legitimate work world, now that he had some agency "muscle" behind him.

Rather than opting out of the case, the psychologist chose an indirect path to help the patient. By deciding to utilize the rehabilitation team as her indirect instrument for intervention, the psychologist was able to affect the patient's rehabilitation experience in a positive manner, while respecting his wish to decline direct psychological services. This approach balances the psychologist's responsibility as a rehabilitation team member with respect for patient autonomy and, secondarily, nonmaleficence.

While these indirect behavioral interventions were not billable in the formal sense, Dr. Morrissey was able to consider her carefully planned consultancy activities as "administrative costs" that enhanced team provision of effective treatment to this patient. Her time-intense contribution to the successful completion of Mr. Snodgrass's rehabilitation program by instrumentally working through the team was attested by her team colleagues. Such a flexible business practice demands collaboration between the psychologist consultant and a creative and committed management team, well versed in the vagaries of serving the rehabilitation needs of individuals who make less-than-desirable choices in the domain of program compliance.

Learning Opportunities

1. Deprived of patient consent to treat, what are some strategies you might employ to ensure psychological needs are met, albeit indirectly?
2. What are some considerations to keep in mind when attempting to adequately inform a patient prior to treatment?

Brief Scenario: Helga Dorfmeier is referred to you for cognitive evaluation related to a recent stroke and questionable decisional capacity. When you meet Helga for the first time as an outpatient, you are struck by her clinical presentation. Her speech is marked by neologisms and dysnomia, resulting in a "word salad," with incomplete comprehension of your communication. Yet, Helga appears determined to communicate discrete messages to you, and is frustrated when she cannot make you understand what seems to her to be clear communication. Helga's husband Bren, who drove her to the appointment, seems to understand at least some of what she is trying to say, but admittedly cannot be sure. Consider how best to preserve patient autonomy within the bounds of her cognitive limitations. How would such a clinical presentation affect the components of your capacity assessment and your interpretation of test results?

Brief Commentary: This patient appears to be demonstrating Wernicke-type aphasia, a detail that was not specifically documented in the medical records accompanying the referral. Comprehension of external communication and the intent of the evaluative consultation remain questions to be addressed regarding **informed consent for assessment**. Assuming that her husband is functioning as Helga's surrogate, does he know the intent and consequences of the evaluation? Essentially, as a surrogate he is representing his wife's wishes regarding submitting to the evaluation. It is likely that if Helga can demonstrate sufficient information processing to participate in the assessment process, the husband/surrogate will need to positively encourage her participation in order to provide her reassurance and external validation of her efforts, at least during the initial portion of the assessment. It can be useful to the clinician for family members to initially support challenging assessment, but only if there is no direct or indirect assistance with responding provided in the support process. The support can then be weaned during the assessment process.

As the rehabilitation psychologist assembles the assessment instruments, the following clinical questions can guide the evaluation and instrument selection. First, is the patient capable of following and remembering explicit instructions for test instruments? This challenge may require clinical evaluation geared to determine the parameters of comprehension—for example, following commands graded from simple to multistep/complex, producing responses that are reliably interpretable, and ability to use alternative forms of responding in lieu of impaired verbalizations (printed words, visual symbols, gestures, etc.). If the patient is able to respond in a consistent manner with reasonable accuracy, the clinician can then select test instruments that **accommodate patient limitations** (Caplan & Shechter, 1995) and address criteria for **capacity evaluation** put forth by Wirshing et al. (1998) and Applebaum (2007).

However, if Helga is not able to respond in a manner indicative of decisional capacity either during clinical or testing evaluation, her husband would be expected to serve as her decision-making surrogate. In such instances, the surrogate is expected to consider components of decisions under the ethics concept of **substituted judgment**. This concept involves the surrogate making decisions as the patient would if capacitated. It is crucially important that potential surrogate decision-makers have a thorough knowledge of the beliefs and values of the individual whom they would represent in case of incapacity.

RELEVANT ETHICS STANDARDS

3.10 Informed Consent
9.01 (a, c) Bases of Assessments
9.02 (b, c) Use of Assessments
9.03 (a 3) Informed Consent in Assessments
9.06 Interpreting Assessment Results
9.10 Explaining Test Results

7 Conclusions

WE HAVE ENDEAVORED to present ethics case discussion and analysis material in a manner that evokes interest in pursuing contextual factors that influenced the events portrayed in the course of arriving at alternative solutions. This emphasis on contextual background is born of the authors' experience in applied ethics. Several decades of health center ethics committee membership/leadership, teaching ethics courses to budding health care professionals and specialists, and wrestling with clarifying psychologists' vested interests within the evolving bioethics literature have unabashedly influenced our message. Thus, our accrued wisdom is presented for your edification and evaluation.

As you have no doubt noted, several themes emerge from a careful reading of this volume. First is paramount. Given psychologists' extensive training in efficient problem-solving, refraining from jumping directly from the emotionally laden critical incident to resolution is a challenge. Ferreting out the motivations, environmental influences, and psychosocial nuances of the interactions affecting key stakeholders in the scenarios is critical to adequately understanding how the ethical conflict occurred and evolved. In order to create a palette of possible solutions on which all stakeholders can agree to negotiate is no mean task. The role of mediator, armed with contextually relevant information, is tailor-made for rehabilitation psychologists.

Second, the varied roles of rehabilitation psychologists that you have discovered in the case examples are included by design. As we move forward in defining our maturing profession, embracing the array of possible influential roles available to rehabilitation psychologists within the multifaceted health care arena is both a natural process and a mandate. Our training in the "systems approach" to health care provision within the rehabilitation team process allows us to migrate (hopefully) smoothly within and across social-organizational borders and boundaries. Our training in efficient and effective service provision, focused on benefiting those persons served as well as our colleagues, serves to facilitate the process of health care service delivery across the spectrum. However, we must demonstrate our value in order to earn access to the broader system. To the extent that we, as rehabilitation psychologists, expand our view to encompass the professional needs and goals of our peers, we can optimize the relevance of our efforts. In addition, acquiring the reins of leadership and authority within the health care arena requires persistence and the provision of high quality services resulting in measurably positive outcomes.

Finally, we have presented for your intellectual stimulation and enjoyment—yes, enjoyment (a word rarely partnered with the word "ethics")—a methodology for applying the principles and standards of the APA Ethics Code to your unique professional environment. We have discovered that a thorough grounding in the tenets of applied health care ethics facilitates team leadership. Clarity of thought, decisiveness, and solid clinical and social judgment that fall from a practical understanding of the Ethics Code allow rehabilitation psychologists to lead treatment teams by example. We urge you to embrace the Ethics Code as a handbook for everyday clinical, research, consultative, and educational practice, AND to contribute to the serial upgrading of the Code via membership input when survey data are requested by the APA Ethics Committee. Retaining the personal and social relevance of the Code allows it to continue being a living document.

Chapter References

INTRODUCTION

American Psychological Association (APA). (2002). Ethical principles of psychologists and code of conduct. *American Psychologist, 57*(12), 1060–1073. doi: 10.1037/0003-066X.57.12.1060

American Psychological Association (APA). (2006). *APA task force on the assessment of competencies in professional psychology: Final report.* Washington, DC: Author.

American Psychological Association (APA). (2012). Guidelines for assessment of and intervention with persons with disabilities. *American Psychologist, 67*(1), 43–62. Washington, DC: APA Press. doi: 10.1037/a0025892

Beauchamp, T., & Childress, J. (2009). *Principles of biomedical ethics* (6th ed.). New York, NY: Oxford University Press.

Bush, S. (2007). *Ethical decision-making in clinical neuropsychology.* New York, NY: Oxford University Press.

Canadian Code of Ethics. (1991). *Canadian code of ethics for psychologists.* Ottawa, Ontario, Canada: Canadian Psychological Association.

Hanson, S., Guenther, R., Kerkhoff, T., & Liss, M. (2000). Ethics in rehabilitation psychology: Historical foundations, basic principles and contemporary issues. In R. Frank & T. Elliott (Eds.), *Handbook of rehabilitation psychology* (pp. 629–644). Washington, DC: APA Press.

Hanson, S., & Kerkhoff, T. (2007). Ethical decision-making in rehabilitation psychology: Considerations of Latino cultural factors. *Rehabilitation Psychology, 52*(4), 409–420.

Hanson, S., & Kerkhoff, T. (2011). The APA ethical principles as foundational competencies: Applications to rehabilitation psychology. *Rehabilitation Psychology, 56*(3), 219–230.

Hanson, S., Kerkhoff, T., & Bush, S. (2005). *Health care ethics: A casebook for psychologists.* Washington, DC: APA Press.

Hibbard, M., & Cox. D. (2010). Competencies of a rehabilitation psychologist. In R. Frank, M. Rosenthal, & B. Caplan (Eds.), *Handbook of rehabilitation psychology* (2nd ed., pp. 467–476). Washington, DC: APA Press.

Kerkhoff, T., & Hanson, S. (2012). Ethics in health psychology: Expanding horizons. In P. Kennedy (Ed.), *The Oxford handbook of rehabilitation psychology* (pp. 432–452). New York, NY: Oxford University Press.

Kerkhoff, T., Hanson, S., Guenther, R., & Ashkanazi, G. (1997). The foundation and application of ethical principles in rehabilitation psychology. *Rehabilitation Psychology, 42*(1), 17–30.

Kerkhoff, T., Hanson, S., & Swaine, Z. (2010). Ethical challenges in funding treatment and care in traumatic brain injury: An argument for national health insurance. In M. Ashley (Ed.), *Traumatic brain injury: Case management and rehabilitation* (2nd ed., pp. 961–992). Boca Raton, FL: CRC Press.

Roberto, M. (2009). *The art of critical decision making.* Chantilly, VA: The Teaching Company: Master Lectures.

Rodolfa, E., Bent, R., Eisman, E., Nelson, P., Rehm, L., & Ritchie, P. (2005). A cube model for competency development: Implications for psychology educators and regulators. *Professional Psychology: Research and Practice, 38*(5), 452–462. doi: 10.1037/0735-7028.38.5.452

Rogerson, M., Gottlieb, M., Handelsman, M., Knapp, S., & Younggren, J. (2011). Nonrational processes in ethical decision making. *American Psychologist, 66*(7), 614–623. doi: 10.1037/a0025215

Stiers, W., Hanson, S., Turner, A., Stucky, K., Barisa, M., Brownsberger, M.,…Kuemmel, A. (2012). Guidelines for post-doctoral training in rehabilitation psychology. *Rehabilitation Psychology, 57*(4), 267–279. doi 10.137/a0030774

CHAPTER 1

American Psychological Association (APA). (2002). Ethical principles of psychologists and code of conduct. *American Psychologist, 57*(12), 1060–1073. doi: 10.1037/0003-066X.57.12.1060

Bush, S. (2007). *Ethical decision-making in clinical neuropsychology.* New York, NY: Oxford University Press.

Canadian Psychological Association. (1991). *Canadian code of ethics for psychologists.* Ottawa, Ontario, Canada: Author.

Hanson, S., Kerkhoff, T., & Bush, S. (2005). *Health care ethics: A casebook for psychologists.* Washington, DC: APA Press.

Kerkhoff, T., & Pugh, E. (2006). *Ethical decision-making in occupational therapy practice* (Instructional video). Gainesville: University of Florida Department of Occupational Therapy, Distance Learning Program.

Kitchener, K. S. (2000). *Foundations of ethical practice, research, and teaching in psychology.* Mahwah, NJ: Erlbaum.

Koocher, G., & Keith-Spiegel, P. (1998). *Ethics in psychology: Professional standards and cases* (2nd ed.). New York, NY: Oxford University Press.

National Association of Social Workers (NASW). (2012). Essential steps for ethical problem-solving. Retrieved from http://www.socialworkers.org/pubs/code/oepr/steps.asp

Roberto, M. (2009). *The art of critical decision making.* Chantilly, VA: The Teaching Company: Master Lectures.

Rogerson, M., Gottlieb, M., Handelsman, M., Knapp, S., & Younggren, J. (2011). Nonrational processes in ethical decision making. *American Psychologist, 66*(7), 614–623. doi: 10.1037/a0025215

Weber, L. (2001). *Business ethics in health care: Beyond compliance*. Bloomington: Indiana University Press.

CHAPTER 2

American Psychological Association. Ethics Code. (2002). Ethical principles of psychologists and code of conduct. *American Psychologist, 57*(12), 1060–1073. doi: 10.1037/0003-066X.57.12.1060

American Psychological Association (APA) (2010). Ethical principles of psychologists and code of conduct – 2010 Amendments. Retrieved from http://www.apa.org/aspx

American Speech-Language Hearing Association. (2012). *Code of ethics (Rules of ethics, I)*. Retrieved from http://www.asha.org/policy

Anbarci, N., & Coglayan, M. (2005). *Cadaveric vs. live-donor kidney transplants: The interaction of institutions and inequality*. Retrieved from: Anbarci & Coglayan, 2005 http://www.gla.ac.uk/media/media 2005 en.pdf

Beauchamp, T., & Childress, J. (2009). *Principles of biomedical ethics* (6th ed.). New York, NY: Oxford University Press.

Rodrigue, J. R. (2002, May). *Ethical and psychological dilemmas in transplantation*. Invited paper presented at the 10th Annual UNOS Transplant Management Forum, Las Vegas, NV. Personal Communication.

Rosner, F. (2006, August). Living vs. cadaveric organ donors: Ethical, legal and religious considerations. *Annals of Internal Medicine, 145*(3), 157–164.

CHAPTER 3

American Psychological Association. (2002). Ethical principles of psychologists and code of conduct. *American Psychologist, 57*(12), 1060–1073. doi: 10.1037/0003-066X.57.12.1060

Beauchamp, T., & Childress, J. (2009). *Principles of biomedical ethics* (6th ed.). New York, NY: Oxford University Press.

Florida Statutes. *FS 825.102-Abuse, aggravated abuse, and neglect of an elderly person or disabled adult; penalties*. Retrieved from: http://www.lawserver.com/law/state/florida/statutes/__825-102

Fisher, M. A. (2012). Confidentiality and record keeping. In S. J. Knapp, M. C. Gottlieb, M. M. Handelsman, & L. D. VandeCreek (Eds.), *APA handbook of ethics in psychology. Volume 1: Moral foundations and common themes* (pp. 333–375). Washington, DC: American Psychological Association. doi: 10.1037/13271-013

Goodyear, R. K., & Rodolfa, E. (2012). Negotiating the complex ethical terrain of clinical supervision. In S. J. Knapp, M. C. Gottlieb, M. M. Handelsman, & L. D. VandeCreek (Eds.), *APA handbook of ethics in psychology. Volume 2: Practice, teaching, and research* (pp. 261–275). Washington, DC: American Psychological Association. doi: 10.1037/13272-013

Hanson, S., & Kerkhoff, T. (2011). The APA ethical principles as foundational competencies: Applications to rehabilitation psychology. *Rehabilitation Psychology, 56*(3), 219–230.

Health Insurance Portability and Accountability Act of 1996. Retrieved from http://www.hhs.gov/ocr/hipaa/

Kirschner, K., Kerkhoff, T., Butt, L., Yamada, R., Battaglia, C., Wu, J., ... Bahr, E. (2011, October). "I don't want to live this way, Doc. Please take me off the ventilator and let me die." *PM&R*, *3*, 967–974.

National Academy of Neuropsychology. (2000). Test security: Official statement of the National Academy of Neuropsychology. *Archives of Clinical Neuropsychology, 15*(5), 383–386.

CHAPTER 4

American Psychological Association Ethics Code (APA)., (2002). Ethical principles of psychologists and code of conduct. *American Psychologist, 57*(12), 1060–1073. doi: 10.1037/0003-066X.57.12.1060

Weber, L. (2001). *Business ethics in healthcare: Beyond compliance.* Bloomington: Indiana University Press.

CHAPTER 5

American Psychological Association. (2002). Ethical principles of psychologists and code of conduct. *American Psychologist, 57*(12), 1060–1073. doi: 10.1037//0003-066X.57.12.1060

Beauchamp, T., & Childress, J. (2009). *Principles of biomedical ethics* (6th ed.). New York, NY: Oxford University Press.

Emanuel, E. (2004). Ending concerns about undue inducement. *Journal of Law, Medicine and Ethics, 32*, 100–115.

Halpern, S. D., Karlawish, J. H. T., Casarett, D., Berlin, J. A., & Asch, D. A. (2004). Empirical assessment of whether moderate payments are undue or unjust inducements for participation in clinical trials. *Archives of Internal Medicine, 164*(7), 801–803. doi: 10.1001/archinte.164.7.801

Sieber, J. E. (2012). Research with vulnerable populations. In S. J. Knapp, M. C. Gottlieb, M. M. Handelsman, & L. D. VandeCreek (Eds.), *APA handbook of ethics in psychology. Volume 2: Practice, teaching, and research* (pp. 371–384). Washington, DC: American Psychological Association. doi: 10.1037/13272-017

Singer, E., & Couper, M. P. (2008). Do incentives exert undue influence on survey participation? Experimental evidence. *Journal of Empirical Research on Human Research Ethics, 3*(3): 49–56. doi:10.1525/jer.2008.3.3.49

US Code of Federal Regulations. (2003). *Common rule for the protection of human subjects.* 45 CFR 46.116.

CHAPTER 6

American Psychological Association. (2002). Ethical principles of psychologists and code of conduct. *American Psychologist, 57*(12), 1060–1073. doi: 10.1037/0003-066X.57.12.1060

Applebaum, P. (2007). Assessment of patients' competence to consent to treatment. *New England Journal of Medicine, 357*, 1834–1840.

Beauchamp, T., & Childress, J. (2009). *Principles of biomedical ethics* (6th ed.). New York, NY: Oxford University Press.

Bush v. Schiavo, 2004 Fla, Lexis 1539 (Fla., September 23, 2004).

Canterbury v. Spence, 464 F.2d 772 (D.C. Cir. 1972).

Caplan, B., & Shechter, J. (1995). The role of neuropsychological assessment in rehabilitation:

History, rationale and examples. Chapter in L. A. Cushman & M. J. Scherer (Eds.), *Psychological Assessment in Medical Rehabilitation* pp. 359–392). Washington, DC: APA Press.

Hanson, S., & Kerkhoff, T. (2004). The implications of bioethical principles in traumatic brain injury. In M. Ashley (Ed.), *Traumatic brain injury: Rehabilitation and case management (pp. 685–726)*. Boca Raton, FL: CRC Press.

Knapp, S. J., & Gavazzi, J. (2012). Ethical issues with patients at a high risk for treatment failure. In S. J. Knapp, M. C. Gottlieb, M. M. Handelsman, & L. D. VandeCreek (Eds.), *APA handbook of ethics in psychology. Volume 1: Moral foundations and common themes* (pp. 401–415). Washington, DC: American Psychological Association. doi: 10.1037/13271-015.

Quill, T. (2005). Terri Schiavo—A tragedy compounded. *New England Journal of Medicine, 352*, 1630–1633.

Schindler Schiavo v. Schiavo, 2005 Fla, No. 0511556, D.C. Docket no. CV-05-00530-T (Appeal from the US District Court of the Middle District of Florida, March 23, 2005).

Weber, L. (2001). *Business ethics in health care: Beyond compliance*. Bloomington: Indiana University Press

Wirshing, D. A., Wirshing, W. C., Marder, S. R., Liberman, R. P., & Mintz, J. (1998). Informed consent: Assessment of comprehension. *American Journal of Psychiatry, 155*(11), 1508–1511.

Additional Readings and Resources

The reader interested in pursuing more in-depth information regarding applied ethics relevant to rehabilitation psychologists in their varied roles as clinicians, consultants, educators, and researchers will find this appendix useful. The material is organized in sections around topical content, and represents a wide-ranging compendium of health care ethics issues, with formats including both research studies and commentary. The literature sampled extends beyond the immediate rehabilitation treatment and research environments, in order to apprise the reader of ethics issues that affect the whole of health care.

The authors are committed to the concept of the biopsychosocial model as fundamental to all aspects of health care. Rehabilitation psychologists have traditionally been at the forefront of conceptualizing health care in this multimodal, interactive, and interleaved manner. Therefore, the wide-ranging array of topics will be somewhat familiar to our specialty. We endeavor to present more recent literature in this chapter, as bioethics is a field that both parallels and reflects the evolution of worldwide systems of health care.

THE TOPICAL CONTENT SECTIONS INCLUDE:
Bioethics
Capacity/Competence
Competencies in Ethics and Graduate Training
Decision-Making: Ethical and Clinical
Diversity
End of Life Issues
Ethics in Health Care Settings
Ethics Codes—Rehabilitation Professional Disciplines
Legislation/Legal Issues
Organizational Ethics and Decision-Making in Health Care

Patient Autonomy
Patient Responsibilities
Placebo Treatment
Research Ethics
Social Policy
Surrogate Decision-Making
Technology

BIOETHICS

Beauchamp, T., & Childress, J. (2009). *Principles of biomedical ethics* (6th ed.). New York, NY: Oxford University Press.

Bersoff, D. (2008). *Ethical conflicts in psychology* (4th ed.). Washington, DC: American Psychological Association.

Breslin, J., MacRae, S., Bell, J., & Singer, P. (2005). University of Toronto Joint Centre for Bioethics Clinical Ethics Group, Top 10 health care ethics challenges facing the public: Views of Toronto bioethicists. *BMC Medical Ethics, 6*(5), 49–56. doi: 10.1186/1472-6939-6-5

Dodds, S. (2005). Gender, aging, and injustice: Social and political context of bioethics. *Journal of Medical Ethics, 31*(5), 295–298. doi: 10.1136/jme.2003.006726

Fischback, G., & Fischback, R. (2004). Stem cells: Science, policy and ethics. *Journal of Clinical Investigation, 114*(10), 1364–1370. doi: 10.1172/JCI2004423549

CAPACITY/COMPETENCE

Eastman, N., & Starling, B. (2005). Mental disorder ethics: Theory and empirical investigation. *Journal of Medical Ethics, 32*(2), 94–99. doi: 10.1136/jme,2005.013276

Grisso, T., & Appelbaum, P. (1998). *Assessing competence to consent to treatment: A guide for physicians and other health care professionals*. New York, NY: Oxford University Press.

Werner, P., & Korczyn, A. (2008). Mild cognitive impairment: Conceptual, assessment, ethical, and social issues. *Clinical Interventions in Aging, 3*(3), 413–420.

COMPETENCIES IN ETHICS AND GRADUATE TRAINING

Beinart, H., Llewelyn, S., & Kennedy, P. (2009). Competency approaches, ethics and partnership in clinical psychology. In H. Beinart, P. Kennedy, & S. Llewelyn (Eds.), *Clinical psychology in practice* (pp. 18–32). Leicester, England: British Psychological Society.

Hanson, S., & Kerkhoff, T. (2011). The APA Ethical Principles as a foundational competency: Application to rehabilitation psychology. *Rehabilitation Psychology, 56*(3), 219–230. doi: 10.1037/a0024206

Hibbard, M., & Cox, D. (2010). Competencies of a rehabilitation psychologist. In R. Frank, M., Rosenthal, & B Caplan (Eds.), *Handbook of rehabilitation psychology* (2nd ed., pp. 467–475). Washington, DC: American Psychological Association.

Kerns, R., Bery, S., Frantsve, L., & Linton, J. (2009). Life-long competency development in clinical health psychology. *Training and Education in Professional Psychology, 3*(4), 212–217. doi:10.1037/10016753

Klepac, K., Ronan, G., Andrasik, F., Arnold, K., Belar, C., Berry, S.,...Dowd, E. T. (2012). Guidelines for cognitive behavioral training within doctoral psychology programs in the United States: Report of the inter-organizational task force on cognitive and behavioral psychology doctoral education. *Behavior Therapy, 43*, 687–697. doi: 10.1016/j.beth.2012.05.002. Accessed from www.sciencedirect.com

DECISION-MAKING: ETHICAL AND CLINICAL

Blackmer, J. (2001). Tube feeding in stroke patients: A medical and ethical perspective. *Canadian Journal of Neurological Science, 28*(2), 101–106.

Bush, S. (2007). *Ethical decision making in clinical neuropsychology*. Oxford Workshop Series. New York, NY: Oxford University Press.

Hurst, S., Hull, S., DuVal, G., & Danis, M. (2005). How physicians face ethical difficulties: A qualitative analysis. *Journal of Medical Ethics, 31*(1), 7–14. doi: 10.1136/jme.2003.005835

Kaldjian, L., Jones, E., Wu, B., Forman-Hoffman, V., Levi, B., & Rosenthal, G. (2007). Disclosing medical errors to patients: Attitudes and practices of physicians and trainees. *Society of General Internal Medicine, 22*(7), 988–996. doi: 10.1007/s11606-007-0227-z

Mukherjee, D., Levin, R., & Heller, W. (2006). The cognitive, emotional, and social sequelae of stroke: Psychological and ethical concerns in post-stroke adaptation. *Topics in Stroke Rehabilitation, 13*(4), 26–35. doi: 10.1310/tsr1304-26

Petrova, M., Dale, J., & Fulford, B. (2006). Values-based practice in primary care: Easing the tensions between individual values, ethical principles and best evidence. *British Journal of General Practice, 56*, 703–709. PMCID: PMC1.

Reed, A., Mikels, J., & Simon, K. (2008). Older adults prefer less choice than younger adults. *Psychology of Aging, 23*(3), 671–675. doi: 10.1037/a0012772

Stein, J., & Wagner, L. (2006). Is informed consent a "Yes or No" response? Enhancing the shared decision-making process for persons with aphasia. *Topics in Stroke Rehabilitation, 13*(4), 42–46. doi: 10.1310/tsr1304-42

Thornton, T. (2006). Tacit knowledge as the underlying factor in evidence based medicine and clinical judgment. *Philosophy, Ethics and Humanities in Medicine, 1*(2), 1–10. doi: 10.1186/1747-5341-1-2

Torke, A., & Sachs, G. (2008). Self-neglect and resistance to intervention: Ethical challenges for clinicians. *Journal of General Internal Medicine, 23*(11), 1926–1927. doi: 10.1007/s11606-008-0807-6

van Til, J., Drossaert, C., Punter, A., & Ijzerman, M. (2010). The potential for shared decision-making and decision aids in rehabilitation medicine. *Journal of Rehabilitation Medicine, 42*, 598–604. doi:10.2340/16501977-0549

Wagner, L., & Stein, J. (2006). Failure to achieve assent in a communicative patient: What are the caregiver's obligations? *Topics in Stroke Rehabilitation, 13*(4), 36–41. doi: 10.1310/tsr1304-36

DIVERSITY

Cochran, P., Marshall, C., Garcia-Downing, C., Kendall, E., Cook, D., McCubbin, L., & Glover, R. (2008). Indigenous ways of knowing: Implications for participatory research and community. *American Journal of Public Health, 98*, 22–27. doi: 10.2105/AJPH.2006.093641

Gallardo M., Johnson, J., Parham, T., & Carter, J. (2009). Ethics and multiculturalism:

Advancing cultural and clinical responsiveness. *Professional Psychology: Research and Practice, 40*(5), 425–435. doi: 10.1037/a0016871

Hanson, S., & Kerkhoff, T. (2007). Ethical decision-making in rehabilitation: Consideration of Latino cultural factors. *Rehabilitation Psychology, 52*(4), 409–420. doi: 10.1037/0090-5550.52.4.409

Humayun, A., Fatima, N., Naqqash, S., Hussain, S., Rasheed, A., Imtiaz, H., & Imam, S. (2008). Patients' perception and actual practice of informed consent, privacy and confidentiality in general medical outpatient departments of two tertiary care hospitals of Lahore. *BMC Medical Ethics, 9*, 14. doi: 10.1186/1472-6939-9-14

Kostopoulou, V., & Katsouyanni, E. (2006). The truth-telling issue and changes in lifestyle in patients with cancer. *Journal of Medical Ethics, 32*(12), 693–697. doi: 10.1136/jme.2005.01.5487

Reger, M., Etherage, J., Reger, G., & Gham, G. (2008). Civilian psychologists in an army culture: The ethical challenge of cultural competence. *Military Psychology, 20*, 21–35. doi: 10.1080/08995600701753144

Stuart, R. (2004). Twelve practical suggestions for achieving multicultural competence. *Professional Psychology: Research and Practice, 35*(1), 3–9. doi 10.1037/0735-7028.35.1.3

Tekola, F., Bull, S., Farsides, B., Newport, J., Adeyemo, A, Rotimi, C., & Davey, G. (2009). Impact of social stigma on the process of obtaining informed consent for genetic research on podoconiosis: A qualitative study. *BMC Medical Ethics, 10*, 13. doi: 10.1186/1472-6939-10-3

Westra, A., Willems, D., & Smit, B. (2009). Communicating with Muslim parents: "The four principles" are not as culturally neutral as suggested. *European Journal of Pediatrics, 168*, 1383–1387. doi: 10.1007/s00431-009-0970-8

END OF LIFE ISSUES

Chapple, A., Ziebland, S., McPherson, A., & Herxheimer, A. (2006). What people close to death say about euthanasia and assisted suicide: A qualitative study. *Journal of Medical Ethics, 32*, 706–710. doi: 10.1136/jme.2006.015883

Rydvall, A., & Lynde, N. (2008). Withholding and withdrawing life-sustaining treatment: A comparative study of the ethical reasoning of physicians and the general public. *Critical Care, 12*, R13. doi: 10.1186/cc6786

Visser, A., Dijkstra, G., Kuiper D., de Jong, P., Franssen, C., Gansevoort R., et al. (2009). Accepting or declining dialysis: Considerations taken into account by elderly patients with end-stage renal disease. *Journal of Nephrology, 22*(6), 794–799.

ETHICS IN HEALTH CARE SETTINGS

Hanson, S., & Kerkhoff, T. (2010). Ethics. In R. G. Frank, M. Rosenthal, & B. Caplan (Eds.), *Handbook of rehabilitation psychology* (pp. 427–437). Washington, DC: APA Press.

Hanson, S., & Kerkhoff, T. (2011). The health care setting: Implications for ethical psychology practice. In S. Knapp (Ed.), *APA handbook of ethics in psychology: Vol. 1. Moral foundations and common themes* (pp. 75–89). Washington, DC: American Psychological Association.

Hanson, S., Kerkhoff, T., & Bush, S. (2005). *Health care ethics: A casebook for psychologists.* Washington, DC: APA Press.

ETHICS CODES—REHABILITATION PROFESSIONAL DISCIPLINES

American Medical Association Council on Ethical and Judicial Affairs. (2010). *Code of medical ethics of the American Medical Association: 2010–2011 Edition*. Chicago, IL: American Medical Association.

American Nurses Association. (2001). *Code of ethics for nurses*. Retrieved from http://www.nursingworld.org/MainMenuCategories/EthicsStantards/CodeofEthicsforNurses.aspx

American Occupational Therapy Association. (2010). Occupational therapy code of ethics and ethics standards. *American Journal of Occupational Therapy, 64*(November/December Supplement), 1–11.

American Psychological Association. (2002). Ethical principles of psychologists and code of conduct. *American Psychologist, 57*(12), 1060–1073. doi: 10.1037–0003–066X.57.12.1060

American Psychological Association. (2002, 2010). *Ethical principles of psychologists and code of conduct* (2010 Amendments). Retrieved from http://www.apa.org/print-this.aspx

American Speech-Language Hearing Association. (2010). *Code of ethics*. Retrieved from http://www.asha.org/policy

National Association of Social Workers. (2008). *Code of ethics of the National Association of Social Workers (Revised). Retrieved from* http://www.naswdc.org/pubs/code/code.asp

Swisher, L., & Hiller, P. (2010). The revised APTA code of ethics for the physical therapist and standards of ethical conduct for the physical therapy assistant: Theory, purpose, process, and significance. *Physical Therapy, 90*(5), 803–824.

LEGISLATION/LEGAL ISSUES

Americans with Disabilities Act—1990. Retrieved from http://www.ada.gov

NOTE: The above federal legislation analogously refers to individuals with disabilities experiencing "bothering, tormenting, troubling, ridiculing or coercing because of a disability." The intensity of such behavior needs to be severe or pervasive in terms of evidentiary proof. This legislation applies to schools, the workplace, and places of public accommodation. It does not apply to the home.

Civil Rights Act of 1964, PL 82-352 (78 Stat. 241). Retrieved from http://www.archives.gov/education/lessons/covil-rights-act/ 9/16/2011

NOTE: Title VII of this legislation created the Equal Employment Opportunity Commission (EEOC), which is the enforcement arm of the law. Federal law pertaining to potential abuse of individuals with disabilities may be argued under the concepts of intimidation or harassment in the workplace.

Compilation of Patient Protection and Affordable Care Act (PL 111-148, 5/2010). Retrieved from http://docs.house.gov/energycommerce/ppacacon.pdf

Federal Patient Self-Determination Act 1990. Sec. 4751. *Requirements for advance directives under state plans for medical assistance.* 42 U.S.C. 1395 cc (a)

Florida State Statute, Title XLVI, Chapter 825, Retrieved from: http://www.leg.state.fl.us/Statutes/index.cfm?App_mode=Display_Statute&URL=0800-0899/0825/0825Contentsindex.html&StatuteYear=2011&Title=%2D%3E2011%2D%3EChapter%20825

NOTE: The above is an example of state statute addressing the issue of defining and specifying sanctions regarding abuse of individuals with disability.

Health Insurance Portability and Accountability Act (HIPAA, 1996). Retrieved from http://www.hhs.gov/ocr/hipaa

Posgar, G. (2012). *Legal aspects of health care administration* (11th ed.). Sudbury, MA: Jones & Bartlett.

Quill, T. (2005). Terri Schiavo—A tragedy compounded. *New England Journal of Medicine, 352*, 1630–1633.

Rehabilitation Act of 1973 (29 U.S.C. 791 et seq., Section 504). Retrieved from http://users.aristotle.net/~hantley/hiedleg/statutes/rehab73.htm

NOTE: The above federal legislation analogously refers to abuse of individuals with disability as the experience of those persons subject to intimidation and/or harassment. It is expected that state statutes specify enforcement of such legal concepts to citizens.

ORGANIZATIONAL ETHICS AND DECISION-MAKING IN HEALTH CARE

Corrigan, J., Kohn, L., & Donaldson, M. (1999). *To err is human: Building a safer health system.* Washington, DC: Institute of Medicine.

Gawande, A. (2009). *The checklist manifesto: How to get things right.* New York, NY: Metropolitan Books, Henry Holt.

National Institutes of Health. (2008). *Protecting human research participants.* NIH Office of Extramural Research. Retrieved from: http://phrp.hihtraining.com/index/php

Roberto, M. A. (2009). *The art of critical decision making.* Master Lecture Series. Chantilly, VA: The Teaching Company.

Weber, L. (2001). *Business ethics in health care: Beyond compliance.* Bloomington: Indiana University Press.

PATIENT AUTONOMY

Geller, G., Bernhardt, B., Carrese, J., Rushton, C., & Kolodner, K. (2008). What do clinicians derive from partnering with their patients? A reliable and valid measure of "Personal Meaning in Patient Care." *Patient Education Council, 72*(2), 293–300. doi: 10.1016/j.pec.2008.03.025

Giordano, S. (2005). Is the body a republic? *Journal of Medical Ethics, 31*(8), 470–475. doi: 10.1136/jme.2004.009944

Naik, A., Dyer, C., Kunik, M., & McCullough, L. (2009). Patient autonomy for the management of chronic conditions: A two-component re-conceptualization. *American Journal of Bioethics, 9*(2), 23–30. doi: 10.1080/15265160802654111

Stenson, K., Chen, D., Tansey, K., Kerkhoff, T., Butt, L., Gallegos, A., & Kirschner, K. (2010). Informed consent and Phase 1 research in spinal cord injury. *Physical Medicine and Rehabilitation, 2*, 664–670. doi: 10.1016/j.pmrj.2010.05.014

PATIENT RESPONSIBILITIES

Buetow, S., & Elwyn, G. (2006). Are patients morally responsible for their errors? *Journal of Medical Ethics, 32*, 260–262. doi: 10.1136/jme.2005.012245

Evans, H. (2007). Do patients have duties? *Journal of Medical Ethics, 33*, 689–694. doi: 10.1136/jme.2007.021188

PLACEBO TREATMENT

Chung, S., Price, D., Verne, G., & Robinson, M. (2007). Revelation of a personal placebo response: Its effects on mood, attitudes and future placebo responding. *Pain, 132*, 281–288. doi: 10.1016/j.pain.200701.034

Fregni, F., Imamura, M., Chien, H., Lew, H., Boggio, P., Kaptchuk, T., Riberto M., et al. (2010). Challenges and recommendations for placebo controls in randomized trials in physical and rehabilitation medicine. *American Journal of Physical Medicine and Rehabilitation, 89*(2), 160–172. doi: 10.1097/PHM.0b013e3181bc0bbd

Keefe, F., Abernethy, A., Wheeler, J., & Affleck, G. (2008). Don't ask, don't tell? Revealing placebo responses to research participants and patients. *Pain, 135*(3), 213–214. doi: 10.1016/j.pain.2008.01.009

Kermen, R., Hickner, J., Brody, H., & Hasham, I. (2010). Family physicians believe the placebo effect is therapeutic, but often use real drugs as placebos. *Family Medicine, 42*(9), 636–642.

RESEARCH ETHICS

Blackmer, J. (2003). The unique ethical challenges of conducting research in the rehabilitation medicine population. *BMC Medical Ethics, 4*, 2. doi: 10.1186/1472-6939-4-2

Dubois, J. (2008). Hidden data for research ethicists: An introduction to the concept and a series of papers. *Journal of Empirical Research Human Research Ethics, 3*(3), 3–5. doi: 10.1525/jer.2008.3.3.3

Enoch, M., Johnson, K., George, D., Schumann, G., Moss, H., Kranzler, H., & Goldman, D. (2009). Ethical considerations for administering alcohol or alcohol cues to treatment-seeking alcoholics in a research setting: Can the benefits to society outweigh the risks to the individual? *Alcohol Clinical Experimental Research, 33*(9), 1508–1512. doi: 10.1111/j.1530-0277.2009.00988.x

Fries, J., & Krishnan, E. (2004). Equipoise, design bias, and randomized controlled trials: The elusive ethics of new drug development. *Arthritis Research and Theory, 6*(3), R250–R255. doi: 10.1186/ar1170

Helgesson, G., Ludvigsson, J., & Gustafsson-Stolt, U. (2005). How to handle informed consent in longitudinal studies when participants have a limited understanding of the study. *Journal of Medical Ethics, 31*(11), 670–673. doi: 10.1136/jme.2004.009274

Knifed, E., Lipsman, N., Mason, W., & Bernstein, M. (2008). Patients' perceptions of the informed consent process for neurooncology clinical trials. *Neuro-Oncology, 10*(3), 348–354. doi: 10.1215/15228517-2008-007

NIH Office of Extramural Research. *Protecting human research participants.* Retrieved from http://phrp.nihtraining/users/login.php

Shaughnessy, M., Beidler, S., Gibbs, K., & Michael, K. (2007). Confidentiality challenges and good clinical practices in human subjects research: Striking a balance. *Topics in Stroke Rehabilitation, 14*(2), 1–4. doi: 10.1310/tsr1402-1

Wager, E., & Kleinert, S. (2011). Responsible research publication: International standards for authors. A position statement developed at the 2nd World Conference on Research Integrity, Singapore, July 22–24, 2010. In T. Mayer & N. Steneck (Eds.), *Promoting research integrity in a global environment* (pp. 309–316). Singapore: Imperial College Press/World Scientific.

SOCIAL POLICY

Halpern, A., Halpern, J., & Doherty, S. (2008). "Enhanced" interrogation of detainees: Do psychologists and psychiatrists participate? *Philosophy, Ethics and Humanities in Medicine, 3*, 21. doi: 10.1186/1747-5341-3-21

International Association of Applied Psychology. (2008). Universal declaration of ethical principles for psychologists. Retrieved from: http://www.am.org/iupsys/resources/ethics/univ-decl2008.html

Li, L., Wu, Z., Wu, S., Lee, S., Rotheram-Borus, M., Detels, R.,...Sun, S. (2007). Mandatory HIV testing in China: The perception of health-care providers. *Journal of STD AIDS, 18*(7), 476–481. doi: 10.1258/095646207781147355

Mamhidir, A., Kihlgren, M., & Sorlie, V. (2007). Ethical challenges related to elder care: High-level decision-makers' experiences. *BMC Medical Ethics, 8*, 3. doi: 10.1186/1472-6939-8-3

Seker, B., Goldenberg, M., Gibson, B., Wagner, F., Parke, B., Breslin, J., Thompson, A., et al. (2006). Just regionalisation: Rehabilitating care for people with disabilities and chronic illnesses. *BMC Medical Ethics, 7*, 9. doi: 10.1186/1472-6939-7-9

Shostak, S., & Ottman, R. (2006). Ethical, legal and social dimensions of epilepsy genetics. *Epilepsia, 47*(10), 1595–1602. doi: 10.1111/j1528-1167.2006.00632.x

SURROGATE DECISION-MAKING

Berger, J., DeRenzo, E., & Schwartz, J. (2008). Surrogate decision making: Reconciling ethical theory and clinical practice. *Annals of Internal Medicine, 149*(1), 48–53.

Braun, U., Naik, A., & McCullough, L. (2009). Reconceptualizing the experience of surrogate decision-making: Report vs. genuine decisions. *Annals of Family Medicine, 7*(3), 249–253. doi: 10.1370/afm.963

Dunn, M., Clare, I., & Holland, A. (2008). Substitute decision-making for adults with intellectual disabilities living in residential care: Learning through experience. *Health Care Analysis, 16*(1), 52–64. doi: 10.1007/s10728-007-0053-9

TECHNOLOGY

Brashler, R., Savage, T., Mukherjee, & Kirschner, K. (2007). Feeding tubes: Three perspectives. *Topics in Stroke Rehabilitation, 14*(6), 74–77. doi: 10.1310/tsr1406-74

Demiris, G., Oliver, D. P., Giger, J., Skubic, M., & Rantz, M. (2009). Older adults' privacy considerations for vision based recognition methods of eldercare applications. *Technology and Health Care, 17*, 41–48. doi: 10.3233/THC-2009-0530

Glueckauf, R. (2007). Telehealth and older adults with chronic illness: New frontiers for research and practice. *Clinical Gerontologist, 31*, 1–4. doi: 10.1300/J018v31n01_01

Gorini, A., Gagglioli, A., Vigna, C., & Riva, G. (2008). A second life for eHealth: Prospects for the use of 3-D virtual worlds in clinical psychology. *Journal of Medical Internet Research, 10*(3), e21. doi: 10.2196/jmir.1029

Hoffman, H., Doctor, J., Patterson, D., Carrougher, G., & Furness T., III, (2000). Virtual reality as an adjunctive pain control during burn wound care in adolescent patients. *Pain, 85*(1–2), 305–309. doi: 10.1016/S0304-3959(99)00275-4

Lange, A., & Ruwaard, J. (2010). Ethical dilemmas in online research and treatment of sexually abused adolescents. *Journal of Medical Internet Research, 12*(5), e58. doi: 10.2196/jmir.1455

Lustria, M., Cortese, J., Noar, S., & Glueckauf, R. (2009). Computer-tailored health interventions delivered over the web: Review and analysis of key components. *Patient Education and Counseling, 74*, 156–173. doi: 10.1016/j.pec.2008.08.023

Murray, S. (2007). Care and the self: Biotechnology, reproduction, and the good life. *Philosophy, Ethics, and Humanities in Medicine, 2*, 6. doi: 10.1186/1747-5341-2-6

Murtagh, M. (2008). A funny thing happened on the way to the journal: A commentary on Foucault's ethics and Stuart Murray's "Care of the self." *Philosophy, Ethics and Humanities in Medicine, 3*, 2. doi: 10.1186/1747-5341-3-2

Rizzieri, A., Verheijde, J., Rady, M., & McGregor, J. (2008). Ethical challenges with the left ventricular assist device as a destination therapy. *Philosophy, Ethics and Humanities in Medicine, 3*, 20. doi: 10.1186/1747-5341-3-20

Rousche, P., Schneeweis, D., Perreault, E., & Jensen, W. (2008). Translational neural engineering: Multiple perspectives on bringing benchtop research into the clinical domain. *Journal of Neural Engineering, 5*(1), 16–20. doi: 10.1088/1741-2560/5/1/P02

Scully, J. (2008). Disability and genetics in the era of genomic medicine. *Nature Reviews Genetics, 9*, 797–802. doi: 10.1038/nrg2453

Sharkey, N. (2008). The ethereal frontiers of robotics. *Science, 322*, 1800–1801. doi: 10.1126/science.1164582

Index

Tables are indicated by an italic *t* following the page number.

A

accommodation, 117
accuracy, 71
Accuracy in Reports to Payors (6.06), 64*t*
Accuracy in Teaching (7.03), 62
adaptive approach, 81
Adult Protective Services (APS), 61
advocating for individuals with disabilities, 84
alternative solutions
    in decision-making process, 4–5
    relevant factors in, 1
American Board of Professional Psychology, adoption of cube model, xiii
American Board of Rehabilitation Psychology, adoption of cube model, xiii
American Psychological Association (APA), ethics code of. *see* APA Ethics Code
APA. *See* American Psychological Association
APA Ethics Code
    in decision-making process, 3–4
    as enforceable standards, xi
    as foundation of predoctoral competency, xiv–xv
    practical understanding of, 119
    1.02 Conflicts Between Ethics and Law, 64*t*, 96

1.03 Conflicts Between Ethics and Organizational Demands, 20*t*, 71
1.04 Informal Resolution of Ethical Violations, 71, 85, 96
1.08 Unfair Discrimination against Complainants and Respondents, 85
2.01 Boundaries of Competence, 30, 34*t*
2.02 Providing Services in Emergencies, 30
2.04 Bases for Scientific and Professional Judgments, 11*t*, 101*t*
2.05 Delegation of Work, 34*t*
3.01 Unfair Discrimination, 75*t*, 96
3.04 Avoiding Harm, 19, 20*t*, 51, 55*t*, 62, 75*t*, 85, 96, 108, 110*t*
3.05 Multiple Relationships, 19, 51, 62, 110*t*
3.06 Conflict of Interest, 19, 51, 71, 75*t*, 96
3.07 Third-Party Requests for Services, 19, 34*t*
3.08 Exploitative Relationships, 51
3.09 Cooperation with Other Professionals, 19, 34*t*, 44*t*, 64*t*, 101*t*, 110*t*
3.10 Informed Consent, 51, 75*t*, 101*t*, 108, 110*t*, 117
3.12 Interruption of Psychological Services, 75*t*
4.02 Discussing Limits of Confidentiality, 96
4.04 Minimizing Intrusions on Privacy, 96

APA Ethics Code *(Cont.)*
   4.05 Disclosures, 20*t*, 55*t*, 64*t*, 96, 108
   4.06 Consultation, 11*t*
   4.07 Use of Confidential Information for Didactic or Other Purposes, 96
   6.02 Confidentiality of Records, 44*t*
   6.04 Fees and Financial Arrangements, 42, 71
   6.06 Accuracy in Reports to Payors, 64*t*
   7.03 Accuracy in Teaching, 62
   7.04 Student Disclosure of Personal Information, 62
   7.06 Assessing Student and Supervisee Performance, 62
   8.00 Research and Publication, 11*t*
   8.02 Informed Consent to Research, 42, 85, 87*t*
   8.04 Client/Patient, Student, and Subordinate Research Participants, 42, 87*t*
   8.06 Offering Inducements for Research Participation, 42, 87*t*
   8.08 Debriefing, 42, 85
   9.01–.03 Assessment, 64*t*
   9.01 Bases of Assessments, 117
   9.02 Use of Assessments, 117
   9.03 Informed Consent in Assessments, 11*t*, 20*t*, 117
   9.04 Release of Test Data, 44*t*, 48
   9.06 Interpreting Assessment Results, 117
   9.10 Explaining Assessment Results, 20*t*, 64*t*, 117
   9.11 Maintaining Test Security, 44*t*
   10.04 Providing Therapy to those Served by Others, 44*t*
   10.10 Terminating Therapy, 20*t*, 55*t*, 75*t*
assent vs. consent, 108
assessments
   Assessing Student and Supervisee Performance (7.06), 62
   Assessment (9.01–.03), 64*t*
   Bases of Assessments (9.01), 117
   Explaining Assessment Results (9.10), 20*t*, 64*t*, 117
   Informed Consent in Assessment (9.03), 11*t*, 20*t*, 117
   Interpreting Assessment Results (9.06), 117
   Use of Assessments (9.02), 117
assisted suicide, 32

autonomy, 97, 116
Avoiding Harm (3.04), 19, 20*t*, 51, 55*t*, 62, 75*t*, 85, 96, 108, 110*t*

B

Bases for Scientific and Professional Judgment (2.04), 11*t*, 101*t*
Bases of Assessments (9.01), 117
beneficence and nonmaleficence
   balanced with privacy, 97
   health care decisions involved, 8–9
   organ transplantation evaluation
      brief commentary, 18–19
      brief scenario, 18
      case analysis summary, 11–12*t*
      commentary, 15–17
      contextual factors, 14–15
      disposition, 17
      learning opportunities, 18
      overview, 9–10
      resolutions, 12–13
   treatment termination
      brief commentary, 29–30
      brief scenario, 28–29
      case analysis summary, 20*t*
      commentary, 26–27
      contextual factors, 23–25
      critical incident, 19–21
      disposition, 27–28
      learning opportunities, 28
      resolutions, 21–23
biopsychosocial model, xv
boundaries and training limitations, 29, 33
Boundaries of Competence (2.01), 30, 34*t*
business relationships, 51

C

Canadian Code of Ethics (1991), 2*t*
cancer prognoses, 28
Canterbury v. Spence, 97
capacity evaluation, 117
case titles
   "But, I can't afford it," 73–85
   "But it's the only available health care," 85–96
   "Consumer-driven health care gone bad," 53–62
   "Didn't you hear me say NO!," 109–117
   "The 11th Hour Consultation," 32–42

"I can't treat my patient," 62–71
"I just want to get outta here!," 99–108
"Magical Thinking: Hope at all costs," 19–30
"Would you believe it broke again?," 9–19
"You want to see my what?," 42–51
charity care. *See* non-reimbursed care
Client/Patient, Student, and Subordinate Research Participants (8.04), 42, 87*t*
clinical psychology education
   Accuracy in Teaching (7.03), 62
   Assessing Student and Supervisee Performance (7.06), 62
   competencies specific to, xiv–xv
   fundamental transformation in, xiii
   role boundaries/conflicts, 33
   Student Disclosure of Personal Information (7.04), 62
codes of ethics. *See* APA Ethics Code; ethics codes
coercion, 41, 86
competence
   Boundaries of Competence (2.01), 30, 34*t*
   determining specifics of, xii–xiii
   in informed decision-making, 97–98
   in professional practice, 28
confidentiality, 31–32, 44*t*, 49, 95, 96
Confidentiality of Records (6.02), 44*t*
conflict of interest, 19, 51, 70, 71, 73, 75*t*, 96
Conflicts Between Ethics and Law (1.02), 64*t*, 96
Conflicts Between Ethics and Organizational Demands (1.03), 20*t*, 71
consent
   vs. assent, 108
   Informed Consent (3.10), 51, 75*t*, 97–98, 101*t*, 105–106, 108, 110*t*, 117
   Informed Consent in Assessment (9.03), 11*t*, 20*t*, 114, 117
   Informed Consent to Research (8.02), 42, 85, 87*t*
   research informed consent, 41
   See also treatment refusal
consultancy contracts, 115
Consultation (4.06), 11*t*
contingency-based decision-making model, 15
contractual requirements, 115
Cooperation with Other Professionals (3.09), 19, 34*t*, 44*t*, 64*t*, 101*t*, 110*t*

costs vs. benefits, 95
critical incidents, identification of, in Hanson, Kerkhoff, and Bush model, 3
cube model, xiii
cultural concerns, 91–92, 98

D

Debriefing (8.08), 42, 85
decision-making
   alternative solutions in, 4–5
   competence in, 97–98
   contingency-based, 15
   contingency-based model, 15
   Hanson, Kerkhoff, and Bush model, 3–6
   importance of contextual factors in, 118
   informed, 51
   key stakeholders in, 1, 4
   models for, 1–3, 2*t*
   non-rational aspects in, 1–2
   paternalistic, 98
   structured approach, 49
   by surrogates, 98, 116–117
   See also impaired decision-making capacity
decision-making rights, 108
Delegation of Work (2.05), 34*t*
denial of care
   brief commentary, 70–71
   brief scenario, 70
   case analysis summary, 64*t*
   commentary, 69
   contextual factors, 66–69
   critical incident, 63
   disposition, 69
   learning opportunities, 69
   resolutions, 65–66
directed dialogue, in decision-making process, 4–5
disabled patients. *See* persons with disabilities
discharge planning
   brief commentary, 61–62
   brief scenario, 61
   case analysis summary, 55*t*
   commentary, 60
   contextual factors, 57–59
   critical incident, 53–54
   disposition, 60–61
   learning opportunities, 61
   resolutions, 54–57

Index

disclosure
    Disclosures (4.05), 20*t*, 55*t*, 64*t*, 96, 108
    mandated, 108
    in placement services, 95
    Student Disclosure of Personal Information (7.04), 62
discrimination, 75*t*, 83–85, 89–91, 95, 96
discriminatory participant selection, 83–85, 89–91
Discussing Limits of Confidentiality (4.02), 96
disposition, evaluation of, 5
dual roles, 62

E

education. *See* clinical psychology education
emergencies, providing services in, 30
ethical breach, 70
ethical obligation, 70
ethical principles, identification of, 3–4
ethical violations, informal resolution of, 71, 85, 96
Ethics Code of American Psychological Association (APA). *See* APA Ethics Code
ethics codes
    as assurance to consumers, xi
    as foundation for professional practice, xv
    See also APA Ethics Code
ethics committees, in decision-making process, 3
Explaining Assessment Results (9.10), 20*t*, 64*t*, 117
Exploitative Relationships (3.08), 51

F

family wishes, honoring, 26–27
fax machines, 49
Fees and Financial Arrangements (6.04), 42, 71
fidelity and responsibility
    health care decisions involved, 31–32
    information release
        brief commentary, 51
        brief scenario, 50–51
        case analysis summary, 44*t*
        commentary, 48–49
        contextual factors, 46–48
        critical incident, 42–43
        disposition, 50
        learning opportunities, 50
        resolutions, 43–46
    role boundaries/conflicts
        assaults on, 32
        brief scenario, 40–42
        case analysis summary, 34*t*
        commentary, 38–39
        contextual factors, 36–38
        critical incident, 33–35
        disposition, 40
        learning opportunities, 40
        resolutions, 35–36
financial arrangements, 42, 64*t*, 71
financial incentives, 70–71
financial limitations. *See* nonreimbursed care
focal moral virtues, xi
functional competencies, xiv

G

ground rules. *See* directed dialogue

H

Hanson, Kerkhoff, and Bush model, 2*t*, 3–6
harm
    Avoiding Harm (3.04), 19, 20*t*, 51, 55*t*, 62, 75*t*, 85, 96, 108, 110*t*
    from inducement to participate, 41
    protect society from a preventable harm, 108
    threat to academic standing, 62
HIPAA regulations, 49, 97
human rights, APA Ethics Code and, 9. *see also* respect for rights/dignity

I

impaired decision-making capacity
    brief commentary, 107–108
    brief scenario, 107
    case analysis summary, 101*t*
    commentary, 105–106
    contextual factors, 102–104
    critical incident, 99–100
    disposition, 106–107
    learning opportunities, 107
    resolutions, 100–102
inability to pay. *See* non-reimbursed care
incentive policies, 70–71
indigent care. *See* non-reimbursed care
inducement to participate
    brief commentary, 95–96
    brief scenario, 94
    case analysis summary, 87*t*

commentary, 91–93
contextual factors, 89–91
critical incident, 85–86
disposition, 93
learning opportunities, 93
resolutions, 86–89
inequity, 95–96
informal resolution, 70, 84–85
Informal Resolution of Ethical Violations (1.04), 71, 85, 96
information release
  brief commentary, 51
  brief scenario, 50–51
  case analysis summary, 44*t*
  commentary, 48–49
  contextual factors, 46–48
  critical incident, 42–43
  disposition, 50
  learning opportunities, 50
  resolutions, 43–46
informed consent
  for assessment, 114, 116–117
  competence and, 105–106
  as critical to ethical practice, 97–98
  Informed Consent (3.10), 51, 75*t*, 101*t*, 108, 110*t*, 117
  Informed Consent in Assessments (9.03), 11*t*, 20*t*, 117
  Informed Consent to Research (8.02), 42, 85, 87*t*
  See also treatment refusal
informed decision-making, 51
insurance limitations. *See* non-reimbursed care
integrity
  denial of care
    brief commentary, 70–71
    brief scenario, 70
    case analysis summary, 64*t*
    commentary, 69
    contextual factors, 66–69
    critical incident, 63
    disposition, 69
    learning opportunities, 69
    resolutions, 65–66
  discharge planning
    brief commentary, 61–62
    brief scenario, 61
    case analysis summary, 55*t*
    commentary, 60
    contextual factors, 57–59
    critical incident, 53–54
    disposition, 60–61
    learning opportunities, 61
    resolutions, 54–57
  health care decisions involved, 52–53
Interpreting Assessment Results (9.06), 117
Interruption of services (3.12), 75*t*

J

judgment
  Bases for Scientific and Professional Judgment (2.04), 11*t*, 101*t*
  substituted judgment, 117
justice
  balanced with beneficence and nonmaleficence, 10
  health care decisions involved, 71–72
  inducement to participate
    brief commentary, 95–96
    brief scenario, 94
    case analysis summary, 87*t*
    commentary, 91–93
    contextual factors, 89–91
    critical incident, 85–86
    disposition, 93
    learning opportunities, 93
    resolutions, 86–89
  non-reimbursed care
    brief commentary, 84–85
    brief scenario, 83–84
    case analysis summary, 75*t*
    commentary, 80–82
    contextual influences, 78–80
    critical incident, 73–74
    disposition, 82–83
    learning opportunities, 83
    resolutions, 76–77

K

key stakeholders, in decision-making process, 1, 4
Kitchener model, 2*t*
Koocher and Keith-Spiegal model, 2*t*

M

Maintaining Test Security (9.11), 44*t*
mandated disclosure, 108
medical research. *See* research
medico-legal system, in decision-making process, 4

Minimizing Intrusions on Privacy (4.04), 96
minors, 107–108
misdirection of test data, 49
monetary inducements to participate, 41
　See also inducement to participate
motivational sets, of key stakeholders, 1
Multiple Relationships (3.05), 19, 51, 62, 110*t*
multiple relationships of HCPs, 18–19, 50–51, 113

N
NASW model, 2*t*
Non-adherent/noncompliant patients.
　　　See discharge planning; organ
　　　transplantation evaluation; role
　　　boundaries/conflicts
nonmaleficence. *See* beneficence and
　　　nonmaleficence
non-rational aspects, in decision-making process,
　　　1–2
non-reimbursed care
　brief commentary, 84–85
　brief scenario, 83–84
　case analysis summary, 75*t*
　commentary, 80–82
　contextual influences, 78–80
　critical incident, 73–74
　disposition, 82–83
　learning opportunities, 83
　resolutions, 76–77

O
Offering Inducements of Research Participation
　　　(8.06), 42, 87*t*
organizational ethics, 60
organ transplantation evaluation
　brief commentary, 18–19
　brief scenario, 18
　case analysis summary, 11–12*t*
　commentary, 15–16
　contextual factors, 14–15
　disposition, 17
　learning opportunities, 18
　overview, 9–10
　resolutions, 10–14

P
paternalistic decision-making, 98
patient limitations, accommodation of, 117
patient's rights, 31–32
　See also respect for rights/dignity

patient wishes, honoring, 26–27
personal health information (PHI), 49–50
persons with disabilities
　accommodation for, 117
　advocating for, 84
　guidelines for treatment, xi–xii, xiv
　policy application, 95–96
predoctoral competency
　APA Ethics Code as foundation, xiv–xv
　misunderstanding of, 33
privacy, 41, 49, 95, 97
　See also information release
pro bono services. *See* nonreimbursed care
professional judgment, Bases for Scientific and
　　　Professional Judgment (2.04), 11*t*, 101*t*
professional relationships. *See* Cooperation with
　　　Other Professionals; information release
protect society from a preventable harm, 108
Providing Services in Emergencies (2.02), 30
Providing Therapy to Those Served by Others
　　　(10.04), 44*t*

R
raw test data. *See* information release
reasonable person standard, 73
refusal of a key stakeholder, 84
refusal of discharge. *See* discharge planning
rehabilitation psychologists
　broad settings of practice, xv
　competencies specific to, xiv–xv
　foundation for practice, xi–xii
　as mediators, 118
　varied roles of, 118–119
rehabilitation team, in decision-making process,
　　　4–5
relationships
　business relationships, 51
　exploitative relationships, 51
　Exploitative Relationships (3.08), 51
　Multiple Relationships (3.05), 19, 51, 62, 110*t*
　multiple relationships of HCPs, 18–19, 50–51,
　　　113
　See also Cooperation with Other
　　　Professionals; information release
Release of Test Data (9.04), 44*t*, 48
relevant factors, in alternative solutions, 1
requests for services, third-party, 19, 34*t*
research
　Client/Patient, Student, and Subordinate
　　　Research Participants (8.04), 42, 87*t*

Index | 141

inducement to participate
　brief commentary, 95–96
　brief scenario, 94
　case analysis summary, 87*t*
　commentary, 91–93
　contextual factors, 89–91
　critical incident, 85–86
　disposition, 93
　learning opportunities, 93
　resolutions, 86–89
　Informed Consent to Research (8.02), 42, 85, 87*t*
　Offering Inducements for Research Participation (8.06), 42, 87*t*
Research and Publication (8.00), 11*t*
research informed consent, 41
resource allocation. *See* justice
respect for rights/dignity
　health care decisions involved, 97–99
　impaired decision-making capacity
　　brief commentary, 107–108
　　brief scenario, 107
　　case analysis summary, 101*t*
　　commentary, 105–106
　　contextual factors, 102–104
　　critical incident, 99–100
　　disposition, 106–107
　　learning opportunities, 107
　　resolutions, 100–102
　treatment refusal
　　brief commentary, 116–117
　　brief scenario, 116
　　case analysis summary, 110*t*
　　commentary, 113–115
　　contextual factors, 112–113
　　critical incident, 109–111
　　disposition, 115–116
　　learning opportunities, 116
　　resolutions, 111–112
responsibility. *See* fidelity and responsibility
risks of participation (in research), 92–93
role boundaries/conflicts
　assaults on, 32
　brief scenario, 40–42
　case analysis summary, 34*t*
　commentary, 38–39
　contextual factors, 36–38
　critical incident, 33–35
　disposition, 40
　learning opportunities, 40

　resolutions, 35–36
　See also discharge planning

S
self-determination, 97
service termination. *See* non-reimbursed care
social context
　in decision-making process, 4, 9
　of key stakeholders, 1
structured approach, 49
Student Disclosure of Personal Information (7.04), 62
substituted judgment, 117
supervision/consultation, 29–30
surrogate decision-making, 98, 116–117

T
technology, 95
Terminating Therapy (10.10), 20*t*, 55*t*, 75*t*
test data. *See* information release
Third-Party Requests for Services (3.07), 19, 34*t*
"three strikes and you're out" policy, 15, 17
transplant patients. *See* organ transplantation evaluation
treatment
　Providing Services in Emergencies (2.02), 30
　Providing Therapy to Those Served by Others (10.04), 44*t*
　Terminating Therapy (10.10), 20*t*, 55*t*, 75*t*
　See also treatment refusal; treatment termination
treatment non-adherence. *See* organ transplantation evaluation
treatment refusal
　brief commentary, 116–117
　brief scenario, 116
　case analysis summary, 110*t*
　commentary, 113–115
　contextual factors, 112–113
　critical incident, 109–111
　disposition, 115–116
　learning opportunities, 116
　resolutions, 111–112
treatment termination
　brief commentary, 29–30
　brief scenario, 28–29
　case analysis summary, 20*t*
　commentary, 26–27
　contextual factors, 23–26
　critical incident, 19

treatment termination *(Cont.)*
  disposition, 27–28
  learning opportunities, 28
  resolutions, 20–23
trespassing charge, 56, 60
trustworthiness, 62

U

undue inducement. *See* inducement to participate
Unfair Discrimination (3.01), 75*t*, 96
Unfair Discrimination against Complainants and Respondents (1.08), 85

United Network for Organ Sharing (UNOS), options for patients, 16
Use of Assessments (9.02), 117
Use of Confidential Information for Didactic or Other Purposes (4.07), 96

V

violation of trust, 71
vulnerability, 93

W

welfare, 41

About the Authors

Thomas R. Kerkhoff, PhD, ABPP/RP, has spent the past 35 years providing Rehabilitation Psychology services to individuals with varied disabilities. He teaches Ethics at the University of Florida to undergraduate health science majors, along with a doctoral level Rehabilitation Psychology course. He also consults to health care organizations for rehabilitation program development and publishes in the area of applied ethics in health care

Stephanie L. Hanson, PhD, ABPP/RP, received her PhDs in developmental and clinical psychology from Vanderbilt University in 1986 and was one of the first women board certified in Rehabilitation Psychology. She served on the Board of Directors of the American Board of Rehabilitation Psychology for 4 years, and chaired the Ethical and Social Responsibility Committee for APA Division 22 for 7 years. Dr. Hanson is an APA Fellow in Rehabilitation Psychology.

www.ingramcontent.com/pod-product-compliance
Ingram Content Group UK Ltd.
Pitfield, Milton Keynes, MK11 3LW, UK
UKHW041959230426
12048UKWH00008B/433